Fundamentals of
CLINICAL NUTRITION

Roland L. Weinsier, MD, DrPH, FACP

Professor and Chairman, Department of Nutrition Sciences
Professor, Department of Medicine
University of Alabama at Birmingham

ASSISTANT
EDITOR

Sarah L. Morgan, MD, RD, FACP

Assistant Professor
Division of Clinical Nutrition
Departments of Nutrition Sciences and Medicine
University of Alabama at Birmingham

EDITORIAL
CONSULTANT

Virginia Gilbert Perrin

Assistant Editor
Office of University Relations
University of Alabama at Birmingham

*with **57** illustrations, 46 in full color*

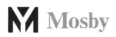 Mosby

St. Louis Baltimore Boston Chicago London Philadelphia Sydney Toronto

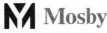 **Mosby**

Dedicated to Publishing Excellence

Publisher: George Stamathis
Editor: Robert J. Farrell
Production Editor: Victoria Hoenigke
Designer: Susan Lane

Cover image: Photomicrography of glycine
© Herb Charles Ohlmeyer/Fran Heyl Associates

Printed in the United States of America

Library of Congress Cataloging-in-Publication Data
Fundamentals of clinical nutrition /   editor, Roland L. Weinsier :
   associate editor, Sarah L. Morgan :   editorial consultant, Virginia
   Gilbert Perrin.
     p.   cm.
   ISBN 0-8016-6571-X : $28.95
   1. Diet therapy. I. Weinsier, Roland L. II. Morgan, Sarah L.
III. Perrin, Virginia Gilbert.
   [DLNM: 1. Diet Therapy. 2. Nutrition. 3. Nutrition Disorders.
WB 400 F981]
RM216.F85 1992
615.8′54—dc20
DNLM/DLC
for Library of Congress   92-48774
                                          CIP

93 94 95 96 GW/VH 9 8 7 6 5 4 3 2

Contributors

Joseph E. Baggott, *PhD*

Assistant Professor
Department of Nutrition Sciences
University of Alabama at Birmingham
Birmingham, Alabama

Charles E. Butterworth, Jr, *MD, FACP*

Professor and General Foods Chair of
    Nutrition Sciences
Department of Nutrition Sciences
University of Alabama at Birmingham
Birmingham, Alabama

Cutberto Garza, *MD, PhD*

Professor and Director
Division of Nutrition Science
Cornell University
New York, New York

Douglas C. Heimburger, *MD, FACP*

Associate Professor and Director
Division of Clinical Nutrition
Departments of Nutrition Sciences and
    Medicine
University of Alabama at Birmingham
Birmingham, Alabama

Judy Hopkinson, *PhD*

Research Instructor
Department of Pediatrics
USDA Agriculture Research Sciences
Children's Nutrition Research Center
Baylor College of Medicine
Houston, Texas

William J. Klish, *MD*

Professor of Pediatrics
Head, Pediatric Gastroenterology
Texas Medical Center
Baylor College of Medicine
Houston, Texas

Yeou-Mei Christiana Liu, *MS, RD*

Instructor
Department of Nutrition Sciences
University of Alabama at Birmingham
Birmingham, Alabama

Kim Bass Mangham, *MS, RD*

Instructor
Department of Nutrition Sciences
University of Alabama at Birmingham
Birmingham, Alabama

A. Kenneth Olson, *MD*

Clinical Assistant Professor
Department of Nutrition Sciences
University of Alabama at Birmingham
Birmingham, Alabama

Howerde E. Sauberlich, *PhD*

Professor and Director, Experimental Nutrition
Department of Nutrition Sciences
University of Alabama at Birmingham
Birmingham, Alabama

Glen Thompson, *PharmD*

Supervisor, Specialty Pharmacy
Department of Pharmacy
University of Alabama Hospital
University of Alabama at Birmingham
Birmingham, Alabama

A. Hal Thurstin, *PhD*

Associate Professor
Department of Psychiatry and Behavioral
    Neurobiology
University of Alabama at Birmingham
Birmingham, Alabama

Acknowledgments

This book is a publication of the Department of Nutrition Sciences and the Clinical Nutrition Research Unit of the University of Alabama at Birmingham. It was supported in part by PHS Grant number PO1-CA28103, awarded by the National Cancer Institute, DHHS and by the National Institutes of Health, Department of Research Resources Clinical Research Center Grant RR-32-31S1.

The chapters entitled "Breastfeeding" and "Nutrition for Infants, Children, and Adolescents" are a publication of the USDA/ARS Children's Nutrition Research Center, Department of Pediatrics, Baylor College of Medicine and Texas Children's Hospital, Houston, Texas. The writing of these chapters was funded in part with federal funds from the U.S. Department of Agriculture, Agricultural Research Service, under Cooperative Agreement number 58-7MNI-6-100. The contents of these chapters do not necessarily reflect the views or policies of the U.S. Department of Agriculture, nor does mention of trade names, commercial products, or organizations imply endorsement by the U.S. Government.

We deeply appreciate the clerical assistance of Mary Roberts, Deitra Terry, and Sharon Matlock.

Preface

As a physician-nutritionist, my background includes training in both internal medicine and clinical nutrition. When I began seeking specialization in clinical nutrition about two decades ago, few options were available. So-called nutrition specialists were in reality gastroenterologists, hematologists, or pediatricians who just happened to profess some knowledge of nutrition as it related to their field of practice. What was a nutritionist, anyway? What procedures would he or she use? With what organ or body system would he or she be identified? At least one could identify with and imagine the role of the cardiologist, the endocrinologist, or the nephrologist.

But times and medical practice have changed. More than half of the leading causes of death in this country are nutrition related. Half of the health-promoting behaviors recommended by physicians in practice are nutrition related. They include recommendations on type and amount of dietary fat intake, salt consumption, cholesterol intake, and vitamin use. In response to the rapidly growing need for physicians who are well trained in nutrition as clinicians, researchers, and teachers, more and more residents are looking for and receiving specialization in clinical nutrition. Drs. Morgan, Heimburger, and Olson, contributors to this book, are also clinical nutrition specialists.

Most readers of this book will be medical students and residents in training, and for most of them this book will represent their major exposure to nutrition. Unfortunately, about two thirds of the medical schools in the United States require no formal instruction in nutrition. Whether your school does or not, this monograph should accomplish the following two objectives: (1) it should complement your medical training by emphasizing the relevance of nutrition to your medical practice; and (2) it should heighten your awareness of nutrition as a medical specialty that is vitally important for both disease prevention and the treatment of diseases of essentially every organ system. If this book achieves either of these aims, it has been a worthwhile endeavor.

Roland L. Weinsier, MD, DrPH

Contents

LIFE, DIET, AND DISEASE

1

Diet and Disease Trends

Normal nutrition
Vegetarian diets
Health foods
Vitamin supplementation

American men and women are now living longer than their parents and grand-parents, and most will die of dramatically different diseases. At the turn of the century, the leading causes of death were infectious diseases—pneumonia, tuberculosis, influenza, and diarrhea-producing infections. Today, heart disease, cancer, and stroke account for two thirds of all deaths in the United States. One out of every three Americans will die of coronary disease before age 65. Many others will die of or be disabled by these illnesses and their complications, including kidney disease secondary to hypertension.

Changes in eating patterns parallel these disease trends. Instead of the high-fiber, low-calorie foods once favored, refined starches, sweets, saturated fats, and salt make up a major portion of today's typical American diet. Combined with sedentary life-styles and cigarette smoking, these habits contribute to alarming rates of hypertension, hyperlipidemia, and cancer in the general population.

Although the rise in deaths from chronic illnesses cannot be totally explained by these eating patterns, mounting scientific evidence underscores the direct relationship between diet and health. Recognizing this link, in 1977 the Senate Select Committee on Nutrition and Human Needs set the following dietary goals for the United States:

1. Increase intake of fruits, vegetables, and whole-grain cereals.
2. Decrease intake of meat while increasing use of poultry and fish.
3. Decrease consumption of high-fat foods and partially substitute poly-unsaturated (vegetable) fat for saturated (animal) fat.
4. Substitute nonfat milk for whole milk.
5. Decrease intake of butterfat, eggs, and other high-cholesterol foods.
6. Decrease use of sugar and foods high in sugar.
7. Decrease use of salt and foods high in salt content.

These guidelines have been updated as the 1990 Dietary Guidelines for Americans, which include the following:

1. Eat a variety of foods.
2. Maintain a healthy weight.
3. Choose a diet low in fat, saturated fat, and cholesterol.
4. Choose a diet with plenty of vegetables, fruits, and grain products.

3

Table 1-1   Recommended dietary allowances* Food and Nutrition Board, National Academy of Sciences—National Research Council, revised 1989. Designed for the maintenance of good nutrition of practically all healthy people in the United States

								Fat-soluble vitamins			
Category	Age (years) or condition	Weight† (kg)	(lb)	Height† (cm)	(in)	Pro-tein (g)	Vita-min A (μg RE)‡	Vita-min D (μg)§	Vita-min E (mg α-TE)‖	Vita-min K (μg)	Vita-min C (mg)
Infants	0.0-0.5	6	13	60	24	13	375	7.5	3	5	30
	0.5-1.0	9	20	71	28	14	375	10	4	10	35
Children	1-3	13	29	90	35	16	400	10	6	15	40
	4-6	20	44	112	44	24	500	10	7	20	45
	7-10	28	62	132	52	28	700	10	7	30	45
Males	11-14	45	99	157	62	45	1000	10	10	45	50
	15-18	66	145	176	69	59	1000	10	10	65	60
	19-24	72	160	177	70	58	1000	10	10	70	60
	25-50	79	174	176	70	63	1000	5	10	80	60
	51+	77	170	173	68	63	1000	5	10	80	60
Females	11-14	46	101	157	62	46	800	10	8	45	50
	15-18	55	120	163	64	44	800	10	8	55	60
	19-24	58	128	164	65	46	800	10	8	60	60
	25-50	63	138	163	64	50	800	5	8	65	60
	51+	65	143	160	63	50	800	5	8	65	60
Pregnant						60	800	10	10	65	70
Lactating	1st 6 months					65	1300	10	12	65	95
	2nd 6 months					62	1200	10	11	65	90

*The allowances, expressed as average daily intakes over time, are intended to provide for individual variations among most normal persons as they live in the United States under usual environmental stresses. Diets should be based on a variety of common foods in order to provide other nutrients for which human requirements have been less well defined. See text for detailed discussion of allowances and of nutrients not tabulated.
†Weights and heights of Reference Adults are actual medians for the U.S. population of the designated age, as reported by NHANES II. The median weights and heights of those under 19 years of age were taken from Hamill PW, Drizd TA, Johnson CL, et al: Physical growth: National Center for Health Statistics percentiles, *Am J Clin Nutr* 32:607-629, 1979. The use of these figures does not imply that the height-to-weight ratios are ideal.

5. Use sugars only in moderation.
6. Use salt and sodium only in moderation.
7. If you drink alcoholic beverages, do so in moderation.

Specific recommendations include basing total calorie intake on a balance of 55% to 60% of calories as carbohydrate, 30% as fat, and 10% to 15% as protein. Cholesterol intake should be less than 300 mg per day; salt intake should be no more than 3 g per day. First published in 1941, the U.S. Recommended Dietary Allowances (RDA), detailed in Tables 1-1 and 1-2, have been updated nine times to reflect new information on safe and adequate nutrient intake. Since the RDA for each nutrient takes into account differences in needs among healthy

Table 1-1   Recommended dietary allowances* Food and Nutrition Board, National
Academy of Sciences—National Research Council, revised 1989.
Designed for the maintenance of good nutrition of practically all healthy
people in the United States—cont'd

Water-soluble vitamins						Minerals						
Thia-min (mg)	Ribo-flavin (mg)	Niacin (mg NE)¶	Vita-min B₆ (mg)	Fol-ate (µg)	Vita-min B₁₂ (µg)	Cal-cium (mg)	Phos-phorus (mg)	Mag-nesium (mg)	Iron (mg)	Zinc (mg)	Iodine (µg)	Sele-nium (µg)
0.3	0.4	5	0.3	25	0.3	400	300	40	6	5	40	10
0.4	0.5	6	0.6	35	0.5	600	500	60	10	5	50	15
0.7	0.8	9	1.0	50	0.7	800	800	80	10	10	70	20
0.9	1.1	12	1.1	75	1.0	800	800	120	10	10	90	20
1.0	1.2	13	1.4	100	1.4	800	800	170	10	10	120	30
1.3	1.5	17	1.7	150	2.0	1200	1200	270	12	15	150	40
1.5	1.8	20	2.0	200	2.0	1200	1200	400	12	15	150	50
1.5	1.7	19	2.0	200	2.0	1200	1200	350	10	15	150	70
1.5	1.7	19	2.0	200	2.0	800	800	350	10	15	150	70
1.2	1.4	15	2.0	200	2.0	800	800	350	10	15	150	70
1.1	1.3	15	1.4	150	2.0	1200	1200	280	15	12	150	45
1.1	1.3	15	1.5	180	2.0	1200	1200	300	15	12	150	50
1.1	1.3	15	1.6	180	2.0	1200	1200	280	15	12	150	55
1.1	1.3	15	1.6	180	2.0	800	800	280	15	12	150	55
1.0	1.2	13	1.6	180	2.0	800	800	280	10	12	150	55
1.5	1.6	17	2.2	400	2.2	1200	1200	320	30	15	175	65
1.6	1.8	20	2.1	280	2.6	1200	1200	355	15	19	200	75
1.6	1.7	20	2.1	260	2.6	1200	1200	340	15	16	200	75

‡Retinol equivalents. 1 retinol equivalent = 1 µg retinol or 6 µg β-carotene.
§As cholecalciferol. 10 µg cholecalciferol = 400 IU of vitamin D.
‖α-Tocopherol equivalents. 1 mg d-α tocopherol = 1 α-TE. See text for variation in allowances and calculation
of vitamin E activity of the diet as α-tocopherol equivalents.
¶1 NE (niacin equivalent) is equal to 1 mg of niacin or 60 mg of dietary tryptophan.
Reprinted with permission from *Recommended Dietary Allowances*, ed 10, © 1989 by the National Academy
of Sciences. Published by National Academy Press, Washington, DC.

people, they should not be used to judge individual requirements. (For information on specific nutrients and their roles in metabolism, see Chapters 5
through 8).

NORMAL NUTRITION

Contrary to what is often reported in the popular press, there are no magical
foods. For most people, a prudent diet consists of a variety of foods—fruits,
vegetables, whole grains, dairy products, lean meat, and fish.

Calorie needs vary according to weight, age, gender, and level of physical
activity. In general, adult men need 2300 to 3100 kcal each day; adult women

Table 1-2 Estimated safe and adequate daily dietary intakes of selected vitamins and minerals*

Category	Age (years)	Vitamins		Trace elements				
		Biotin (µg)	Pantothenic acid (mg)	Copper (mg)	Manganese (mg)	Fluoride (mg)	Chromium (µg)	Molybdenum (µg)
Infants	0-0.5	10	2	0.4-0.6	0.3-0.6	0.1-0.5	10-40	15-30
	0.5-1	15	3	0.6-0.7	0.6-1.0	0.2-1.0	20-60	20-40
Children and adolescents	1-3	20	3	0.7-1.0	1.0-1.5	0.5-1.5	20-80	25-50
	4-6	25	3-4	1.0-1.5	1.5-2.0	1.0-2.5	30-120	30-75
	7-10	30	4-5	1.0-2.0	2.0-3.0	1.5-2.5	50-200	50-150
	11+	30-100	4-7	1.5-2.5	2.0-5.0	1.5-2.5	50-200	75-250
Adults		30-100	4-7	1.5-3.0	2.0-5.0	1.5-4.0	50-200	75-250

*Because there is less information on which to base allowances, these figures are not given in the main table of RDA and are provided here in the form of ranges of recommended intakes.

†Since the toxic levels for many trace elements may be only several times usual intakes, the upper levels for the trace elements given in this table should not be habitually exceeded.

Modified with permission from *Recommended Dietary Allowances*, ed 10, © 1989 by the National Academy of Sciences. Published by National Academy Press, Washington, DC.

require 1600 to 2400 kcal to maintain their weight and energy needs. In either case, those calories should come from foods that yield the most nutrients for the fewest calories. Consider that 1 g of carbohydrate or 1 g of protein has 4 calories, whereas 1 g of fat has 9 calories.

The bulk of an average adult's diet should consist of vegetables, fruits, and unrefined starches such as potatoes, corn, beans, whole-grain cereals, rice, and bread. These three food groups contain most of the vitamins and minerals the body needs. Four to 6 ounces each day of meat, fish, or low-fat cheese will provide adequate protein. Dairy foods should be as low in fat as possible, and fats and oils should be limited to 3 or 4 tsp per day.

VEGETARIAN DIETS

With careful planning, completely meatless diets can be consistent with adequate nutrient intake, and they may offer certain health advantages. Vegetarian diets may either totally exclude meat, fish, eggs, and dairy products (vegan) or rely upon fish (pesco-vegetarian), eggs (ovo-vegetarian), or dairy products (lacto-vegetarian) as a source of protein.

Generally, legumes (dried beans, dried peas, and lentils) are combined with grains, nuts, or seeds to provide all essential amino acids. Vitamin B_{12}, which is found only in animal products, may be supplied through tablet supplementation or through fortified soybean products if no animal products are consumed.

Plant-based diets that include one or a combination of dairy products, eggs, or fish can be nutritionally similar to diets containing meats if menus are planned to provide sufficient calories, essential amino acids, and adequate sources of calcium, riboflavin, iron, and vitamins A, D, and B_{12}. Vegetarian diets may lower risk factors for heart disease by lowering serum cholesterol levels, they may help control body weight, and they may reduce the risk of cancer since they tend to be low in fat and high in fiber and β carotene-containing vegetables and fruits. While complementary plant proteins were stressed in the past, it is now felt that an adequate mix of amino acids will be consumed by eating a variety of plant products.

HEALTH FOODS

The terms *organic, natural,* and *health foods* are loosely defined and are often used interchangeably. There is no scientific basis for claiming that organic foods are more nutritious than conventional foods. Food grown by chemical processes do not necessarily differ in taste, appearance, or nutrient content from those that are grown organically.

The Federal Trade Commission has proposed to prohibit use of the term *health food* in advertising because it may fool consumers into thinking that one specific food is the key to good health.

VITAMIN SUPPLEMENTATION

Although the majority of Americans consuming a varied diet do not require vitamin supplementation, such supplements are routinely consumed by one third

Table 1-3 Situations in which vitamin supplements are recommended

1. Pregnancy
2. Infancy
3. High-risk life-styles
   Low socioeconomic status
   Anorexia/starvation
   Some obesity regimens
   Pregnant teenagers
   Vegans
4. Medical conditions which impair nutrient absorption or utilization, or if nutrient needs are increased

to two thirds of the American population. In some subgroups such as the elderly, use of vitamins may be even higher.

Clear indications for vitamin supplementation (listed in Table 1-3) include pregnancy (folate and iron); infancy (iron); and certain high-risk situations such as anorexia nervosa, participation in some weight-loss programs, and a vegan dietary pattern.

Multiple vitamin supplements can be categorized into two groups. It is important to be familiar with the content of these supplements, since not all contain the same vitamins or doses. The categories are as follows:

1. Replacement or supplemental vitamins. These generally contain 50% to 150% of the RDA for the nutrients provided. Replacement vitamins are best used as supplements in patients at risk for the development of vitamin deficiency.
2. Therapeutic vitamins. These should not exceed two to ten times the RDA for the vitamins included. Fat-soluble vitamins generally are present at two times or less the RDA. Therapeutic vitamins should be used for treatment of deficiency states or in situations where absorption and utilization of vitamins are reduced or requirements are increased.

SELECTED READING

American Dietetic Association Reports: Position paper on the vegetarian approach to eating, *J Am Diet Assoc* 77:61-69, Jul 1980.

Barrett S, Knight G. *The health robbers: how to protect your money and your life*, Philadelphia, 1976, GF Stickley.

Committee on Nutrition, American Academy of Pediatrics: Nutritional aspects of vegetarianism, health foods and fad diets, *Pediatrics* 59(3):460-464, 1977.

Food and Nutrition Board, Commission on Life Sciences, National Research Council: *Recommended dietary allowances*, ed 10 rev, Washington, 1989, National Academy Press.

Food and Nutrition Committee, American Health Foundation: *Problem in defining prudent diet options to the consumer and to the industry*, Activities Report No. 1, New York, 1975, American Health Foundation.

Jarvis WT. Food faddism, cultism and quackery, *Annu Rev Nutr* 3:35-52, 1983.

Nutrition Committee, American Heart Association: *A statement for physicians and health professionals: dietary guidelines for healthy american adults*, Dallas, 1986, American Heart Association.

2

Disorders of Nutrition

Obesity
Diabetes mellitus
Diet, hyperlipidemia, and coronary artery disease
Hypertension
Diet and cancer
Nutrition and oral health
Osteoporosis
Nutritional anemias
Eating disorders

OBESITY

Excess weight has been associated with a number of health problems, ranging from hypertension to cancer. Certainly not all obese persons are unhealthy, and health problems are not evenly distributed among all obese people; nevertheless, there is convincing evidence that obesity has an adverse effect on longevity and, other things being equal, the greater the degree of obesity, the higher the death rate.

Factors predisposing to obesity

It is almost certain that obesity is multifactorial and that there are different types of obesity. Although the causes are not completely understood, the net effect is an imbalance of energy intake and expenditure. One of the oldest schemes for classifying obesity divides it into two types: endogenous, which implies internal causes, and exogenous, suggesting external or acquired causes.

Endogenous factors include genetic, endocrine, and metabolic conditions. Obese parents frequently have obese children (Fig. 2-1), suggesting a familial factor. In fact, this reflects the well-established role of heredity in predisposition to obesity but does not rule out the possible role of the family environment or even that of the in utero and immediate postnatal environment on the observed concordance of obesity in identical twins.

Endocrine abnormalities such as hypothyroidism, Cushing's syndrome (adrenal excess), polycystic ovary syndrome (Stein-Leventhal), and insulinoma can cause obesity, but altogether these account for less than about 1% of all cases. Interestingly, the markedly obese person is least likely to have an endocrine disorder. Other abnormalities to consider include hypothalamic lesions involving centers of appetite control and congenital disorders such as the Prader-Willi syndrome (Fig. 2-2).

9

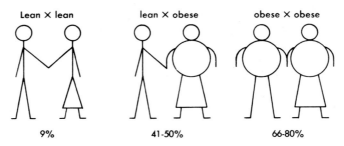

Lean × lean   lean × obese   obese × obese

9%   41-50%   66-80%

Fig. 2-1 Frequency of obesity among offspring of lean and obese parents.

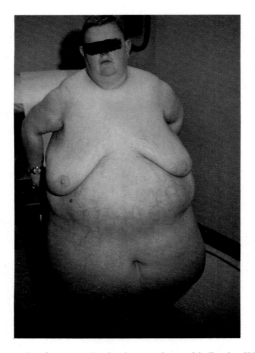

Fig. 2-2 Example of severe obesity in a patient with Prader-Willi syndrome.

Abnormalities or adaptations of energy expenditure may predispose some people to obesity while protecting others. This is suggested by the findings that chronic overfeeding causes less-than-predicted weight gain and that after a meal, obese and previously obese people in some studies have a lower level of energy expenditure than people who were never obese. On the other hand, the resting metabolic rate is generally elevated rather than reduced in the obese person and relative to body size is equivalent to that of the normal weight person. Thus, abnormalities in resting metabolic rate are not likely to explain why obese people maintain their overweight state.

Exogenous factors that may predispose to obesity include dietary excesses, physical inactivity, socioeconomic status, and race. Without question, altered calorie intake can cause weight gain or loss. However, studies of eating behaviors of obese and lean subjects have failed to identify any consistent patterns of calorie intake, eating frequency, or food preferences. In fact, since it is known that the 24-hour energy expenditure in obese people is greater than that in lean people with comparable activity levels, even when greater calorie intake is found in the obese, it does not resolve the issue of whether the high calorie intake preceded or followed the obese state. Physical activity also can influence the energy balance equation, but the question of whether inactivity is the cause or the result of obesity is not answered by findings that obesity is more prevalent among sedentary people and that obese people tend to engage in less exercise than do lean people. Population surveys indicate that obesity is more common among white upper-income men and black lower-income women. These data, too, are descriptive and do not necessarily explain the cause of obesity.

It has been suggested that there are two types of obesity, determined by age of onset and the corresponding proliferation (juvenile onset) or nonproliferation (adult onset) of adipocytes. Although childhood obesity is associated with an increase in the number of fat cells, it now appears that weight gain in later life can also result in proliferation of fat cells as well as simple hypertrophy. Thus, there may not be two distinct forms of obesity according to age of onset.

Diseases associated with obesity

The following diseases and metabolic disorders have been associated with obesity:

- *Osteoarthritis of weight-bearing and non–weight bearing joints.* The occurrence of osteoarthritis in non–weight bearing joints in obese patients suggests that arthritis may not be simply a direct result of mechanical overload.
- *Cancer.* There are high rates of colon, rectal, and prostate cancer in obese men and gallbladder, biliary, breast (if postmenopausal), cervical, uterine, and ovarian cancer among obese women. A possibly important factor relating to cancer of estrogen-responsive organs is the increased conversion in adipose tissue of androgens to estrogens, resulting in elevated estrogen levels.
- *Coronary artery disease (CAD).* Risk of CAD increases with obesity, but it is not clear whether the greater risk is due to the obesity itself or to the presence of concurrent risk factors such as diabetes and hypertension, which are more common among obese people.
- *Diabetes mellitus.* Although not all obese persons become diabetics, it appears that those who are otherwise predisposed to diabetes (e.g., by heredity) are at much greater risk of unmasking the tendency in the presence of obesity.
- *Hepatobiliary disease.* Gallbladder disease, including gallstones, is more frequent in the obese, perhaps because of the increased cholesterol content of bile. Fatty infiltration of the liver also is more likely, particularly with marked degrees of overweight.

- *Hyperlipidemia*. Both cholesterol and triglyceride levels tend to be high in obese persons and to decline as weight is lost. Much of the variability in their levels, however, tends to relate to dietary factors that accompany the obese state or the weight loss program rather than to the degree of adiposity per se.
- *Hypertension*. There is a small but statistically significant association between blood pressure and body weight, although most obese people are not hypertensive. As with lipid levels, blood pressure tends to fall with weight reduction, although the contribution of changes in adiposity per se to blood pressure level is apparently small compared with other factors such as the diet and exercise.
- *Respiratory problems*. Pulmonary hypertension and right-sided heart failure may result from the Pickwickian syndrome (obesity-hypoventilation) caused by marked obesity. This syndrome is characterized by somnolence, hypoxia, and carbon dioxide retention without underlying lung disease.

Body fat distribution may be a better predictor of health hazards of obesity than the amount of body fat. Location of fat stores in the abdominal area (versus the hips and thighs) signals a greater likelihood of diabetes, hypertension, hypertriglyceridemia, ischemic heart disease, and death from all causes.

Guidelines for estimating desirable body weight

The following guidelines may be used to estimate desirable weight for adults:

- *Weight/height tables*. Revisions of the 1959 Metropolitan Life Insurance Company table describe desirable weights as about 5% to 10% higher than previous tables. Since the acceptability of these higher standards is still controversial, the earlier tables (see Table 2-1) are still preferred by many experts. A value of 20% or more above reference weight for height may be considered a health hazard.
- *Body Mass Index (BMI)*. Although less convenient, BMI [weight (kg)/ height (m)^2] is a more accurate estimate of obesity. Obesity is generally defined as a BMI over 25.8 for women and 26.4 for men. These values roughly correspond to 20% above desirable weight for height.
- *Skinfold thickness*. Taken behind the upper arm, below the scapula, or at the waist, this measurement should be about ¼ to 1 inch. To "pinch more than an inch" usually indicates excessive fat reserves.

Prevention and treatment of obesity

Fewer calories and more exercise will produce weight loss, but permanent changes in eating habits and physical activity are required for long-term prevention and treatment of excess weight. A diet program must have a sound scientific rationale, must be safe and nutritionally adequate, and must be practical for long-term use. The program of physical activity must be compatible with the person's life-style in order to result in a permanent increase in activity level. In addition, behavioral or psychological therapy should be a part of the treatment program.

With these points in mind, the following approaches to the treatment of

Table 2-1   Weight-height reference chart (adults)*

| Height (no shoes) | | Reference weight | | | |
| | | Women | | Men | |
Feet/inches	Centimeters	lb	kg	lb	kg
4'10"	147	101	46	—	—
4'11"	150	104	47	—	—
5' 0"	152	107	49	—	—
5' 1"	155	110	50	—	—
5' 2"	157	113	51	124	56
5' 3"	160	116	53	127	58
5' 4"	162	120	54	130	59
5' 5"	165	123	56	133	60
5' 6"	167	128	58	137	62
5' 7"	170	132	60	141	64
5' 8"	172	136	62	145	66
5' 9"	175	140	63	149	68
5'10"	178	144	65	153	69
5'11"	180	148	67	158	71
6' 0"	183	152	69	162	74
6' 1"	185	—	—	167	76
6' 2"	188	—	—	171	78
6' 3"	190	—	—	176	80
6' 4"	193	—	—	181	82

*Data adapted from Metropolitan Life Insurance Company: Build and Blood Pressure Study, 1959. In Weinsier RL, Heimburger DC, Butterworth CE: *Handbook of Clinical Nutrition,* ed 2, St. Louis, Mosby–Year Book, 1989

obesity outline ways to lose weight, but not all are conducive to long-term success.

Weight-loss diets

1. *Novelty diets* include the Beverly Hills, Dolly Parton, Zen-macrobiotic, and the Fit for Life Diet. Weight loss is achieved by limiting food choices and therefore energy intake. The scientific rationale is often unfounded, and documentation of effectiveness and safety is generally unreliable.

2. *Low carbohydrate, quick-weight-loss diets* include the Air Force, Stillman's, and Atkins' diets. The rationale that they produce weight loss by stimulating a fat-mobilizing hormone or by causing significant calorie loss through the ketones excreted in the urine has not been substantiated. Rapid weight loss actually is the result of fluid excretion and is short-lived. Side effects include nausea, fatigue, and increased levels of uric acid and cholesterol.

3. *Very low–calorie diets* include Last Chance, protein-sparing modified fasts, Cambridge, and Optifast. The rationale is that extreme caloric restriction (as low as 300 calories/day) maximizes weight loss, whereas the high protein intake offsets the protein losses of fasting. Protein losses

tend to be less than with fasting but often continue to occur. Unresolved concerns about severe caloric reduction are that losses of lean body, risk of gallbladder disease, and likelihood of weight rebound tend to be greater than with moderate caloric restriction. The safety record of more recent modifications of these diets is better, although long-term effectiveness is still disappointing.

4. *Moderately low–calorie balanced diets* include calorie counting, high fiber or fiber-supplemented approaches, and the time-calorie displacement. Calorie counting is widely used, often with reference to the American Dietetic Association food exchange lists to provide variety in food selection, but data are lacking on the effectiveness and safety. High-bulk diets provide the advantages of slowing the eating rate, reducing calorie absorption, and inducing a feeling of fullness with less food. The EatRight Program used at the University of Alabama at Birmingham incorporates the advantages of both the exchange list approach and the use of high-bulk foods, and it is based on the concept of time-calorie displacement. The spectrum of energy densities of food groups and food selections are shown in Tables 2-2A and B. The typical prescription is for about 1000 kilocalories (kcal)/day eaten as four or more vegetable servings, four or more fruit servings, four starch servings, five meat or dairy servings and three or fewer fat servings each day. The emphasis should be on those foods that require more time to ingest and that are high in bulk and low in caloric density. This program has been shown to be nutritionally adequate, safe, and appropriate for long-term weight control.

Physical activity. The effectiveness of moderate exercise in speeding weight loss is debatable; without diet, it is generally ineffective. However, it may help prevent the muscle and bone loss seen with some low-calorie diets, and it unquestionably improves cardiovascular condition and self-image.

Behavior modification and emotional support. Detailed record keeping of diet, exercise, and emotional factors is important for focusing attention on patterns and problems rather than on pounds. In addition, a successful weight-control program will include learning to eat fattening foods in moderation, thus preventing recurrent feelings of failure from "cheating." In fact, the dietary approach to weight control should emphasize life-long changes in eating patterns rather than temporary use of a diet. The term *diet* implies a time-limited intervention, whereas the major challenge in the treatment of obesity is not weight loss but weight loss maintenance.

Drug therapy. Although appetite suppressants tend to be slightly more effective than placebos in most studies, it is important to be aware that they all have potential adverse side effects, that they should be reserved for certain individuals who need temporary support, and that they do not replace the dietary management and exercise.

Surgical procedures. Surgery is reserved for people who have been at least 100 lb or 100% overweight for three or more years, for people who have serious medical problems related to their obesity, and for those who have failed repeatedly at attempts to lose weight. Commonly used in the past, the jejunal-ileal bypass procedure eliminates about 90% of the absorptive capacity of the bowel, thus causing malabsorption and copious diarrhea. Complications include deficiencies of calcium, magnesium, iron, vitamins A, B_{12}, D, and folate, as well as arthritis, gallstones, liver failure, and kidney disease. Because of these problems, this procedure is no longer considered justifiable.

Stomach-partitioning operations, such as the vertical-banded gastroplasty, reduce the volume of the gastric pouch and reduce the likelihood of overeating. However, voluntary changes in eating behavior are required for the procedure to be effective. Complications are relatively few, but the weight loss is also usually less than with the bypass procedure.

Liposuction is useful for certain individuals who are disfigured due to excessive fat deposition in localized areas. It is important to realize that cosmetic results are variable and that the therapist should be carefully selected on the basis of credentials and experience. Studies have not yet documented a reduction in mortality rates or an increase in life expectancies following surgical therapy for obesity. In addition, complication rates may be high if the procedure is not done by an experienced surgeon.

DIABETES MELLITUS

Diabetes mellitus is the third leading cause of death in the United States. Heredity appears to be a significant factor in its etiology, although the precise genetic factor is unknown. The two major forms of diabetes are type I, insulin-dependent diabetes mellitus (IDDM), and type II, non–insulin-dependent diabetes mellitus (NIDDM).

Symptoms characteristic of uncontrolled diabetes mellitus include increased blood-glucose concentration (hyperglycemia), sugar in the urine (glucosuria), excessive loss of fluids (dehydration), excessive urination (polyuria), thirst (polydipsia), increased appetite and eating (polyphagia), increased blood ketones (ketonemia), ketones in the urine (ketonuria), weakness, weight loss, and vision problems.

Diet is the cornerstone of treatment for both forms of diabetes. The dietary requirements of diabetics differ with the severity of the disease, the type and amount of insulin received, and the amount of activity performed. The most important aspect for the obese diabetic is adjustment of the total calorie intake to attain and maintain desirable body weight. The EatRight Program (described earlier in this chapter) uses a modification of the diabetic exchange guidelines. As described, it uses an approach to change behaviors for long-term weight maintenance.

The diet should be composed of approximately 50% to 60% carbohydrate, 25% to 30% fat, and 15% to 20% protein. The diet must be coordinated with the insulin dosage. Therefore, it is important that the spacing, regularity, and composition of meals and snacks be consistent from day to day. Many insulin-dependent diabetics may be able to maintain blood-glucose control if they eat smaller meals in addition to two or three snacks. Each meal should contain approximately 20% to 40% of the total calories as carbohydrates, and each snack about 10%.

Text continued on p. 20

Table 2-2A   EatRight*

Fat — Eat at most ___ servings‖	45 calorie serving	Meat/Dairy† — Eat ___ servings‖	75 calorie serving	Starch‡ — Eat ___ servings‖	70 calorie serving	Fruit (Fresh, Frozen Sugar-Free)§ — Eat at least ___ servings‖	40 calorie serving	Vegetable (Fresh, Frozen)‖ — Eat at least ___ servings‖ (serving sizes listed are raw vegetables. Cooked vegetables equal ½ cup.)	20 calorie serving
Preferred foods	Serving size	**Preferred foods**	Serving size	**Preferred foods**	Serving size	**Preferred foods**	Serving size	**Preferred foods**	Serving size
Avocado	⅛ med	Fish	1½ oz	**Cooked**		Apples	½ med	Artichoke	½ bud med
Butter		Tuna (water-pack)	2 oz	Beans, cooked		Apricots	2	Asparagus	⅔ c
Regular	1 t	Shellfish		Lentils	⅓ c	Banana	½ sm	Bamboo shoots	½ c
Whipped	1½ t	Crabmeat	3 oz	Kidney	⅓ c	Blackberries	½ c	Bean sprouts	1 c
Cream		Clams	10 med	Lima	⅓ c	Blueberries	½ c	Beets	½ c or 1 med
Half & Half	2 T	Lobster	2½ oz	Pinto	⅓ c	Cantaloupe	¾ c or ⅓	Broccoli	1 c
Sour	1½ T	Oysters	8 med	Soy	¼ c	Cherries, red sweet	11 med	Brussels sprouts	4 med
Whipping	1 T	Scallops	2 oz	White	⅓ c	Cherries, red sour	⅓ c	Cabbage	1 c raw
Nondairy	3 t	Shrimp	20 or 2½ oz	Garbanzo	⅓ c	Grapefruit	½	Carrots	½ c or 1 sm
Cream cheese	1 T	Poultry		Cereal, cooked		Grapes	15	Cauliflower	⅔ c
Margarine		Chicken (no skin)	1½ oz	Buckwheat	½ c	Honeydew	¾ c	Celery (5″)	6 stalks
Diet	1 T	Turkey (no skin)	1½ oz	Millet	½ c	Kiwi	1	Cucumbers	1 lg
Whipped	1½ t			Oatmeal	½ c	Mangoes	½ sm	Eggplant	½ c
Regular	1 t			Whole grain wheat	½ c	Nectarine	1 med		
Mayonnaise									
Regular	1½ t								
Low calorie	1 T								

Nuts, unsalted		Meat		Barley	½ c	Oranges	1 sm	Greens	½ c
Almonds	7	Beef (lean)	1 oz	Bulgar	½ c	Papaya	⅓ med	Green beans	½ c
Brazil	2	Franks (11 g fat)	1	Corn		Peaches	1 med	Green peppers	1 lg
Cashew	4	(count 1 fat)		on cob	3" ear	Pears	½ med	Kohlrabi	½ c
Hickory	7	Pork	1 oz	kernels	½ c	Pineapple	1 sl or ½ c	Lettuce	5 lg leaves,
Peanuts	9	Lamb	1 oz	Peas, black-eyed	⅓ c	Plums	2 med		¼ head
Pecans (halves)	5	Lean luncheon	2 oz	Peas, green	⅔ c	Raspberries	½ c	Mushrooms	7 sm
Walnut (halves)	5	meats (5 g fat)		Potato		Strawberries	10 lg or ¾ c	Okra	½ c,
Oil	1 t	Liver	1½ oz	Baked	1 med	Tangerines	2 sm		6 pods
Peanut butter	1½ t	Veal	1 oz	Boiled	1 med	Watermelon	¾ c	Onions	½ sm
Salad dressing		Sausage (count	1½ oz	Mashed	½ c			Radishes	10 sm
Regular	2 t	1 fat)		Pumpkin	¾ c	**Occasional foods§**		Rutabagas	⅓ c
Low calorie	(see	(see		Rice, brown	½ c			Salad, mixed	1 c
	label)	label)		Squash, winter	½ c	Canned fruit (un-		Scallions	3
Seeds, unsalted		Tofu	½ c	Sweet potato	½ med	sweetened)		Spinach	½ c cooked,
Pumpkin	1 T	Pizza, cheese	1 sl			Applesauce	½ c		1 c raw
Sesame	1 T	(count 1 fat, ½		**Dry**		Fruit cocktail	½ c	Squash, summer	⅔ c
Sunflower	1 T	starch)		Bread, whole	1 sl	Mandarin or-	½ c	Tomatoes	1 sm
Bacon	1 sl	Cheese		grain		anges		Turnips	½ c
Bacon drippings	1 t	Low fat (5 g	1 oz	English muffin,	½				
Cracklings	1 t	fat)		whole grain					
Gravy	2 T	Mozzarella	1 oz						
Salt pork	¼ oz	(part skim)							
		Hard	⅔ oz						

Reprinted with permission of The University of Alabama at Birmingham, c. 1990.

*The spectrum of energy densities of food groups in the EatRight program. Food groups to the right are lowest in energy density, highest in bulk, and require a longer time to eat.

†Weigh portions after cooking.

‡Cooked starches should represent at least half the total intake of starch.

§Up to two items per week.

‖The number of servings to be eaten in each category depends upon the caloric level of the diet prescribed. As commonly used examples: 4 vegetables, 4 fruits, 4 starch, 5 milk/meat, 3 fat servings per day is approximately 1030 kcal/day.

Continued.

Table 2-2A   EatRight—cont'd

Fat — Eat at most ___ servings||		Meat/Dairy† — Eat ___ servings||		Starch‡ — Eat ___ servings||		Fruit (Fresh, Frozen Sugar-Free)§ — Eat at least ___ servings||		Vegetable (Fresh, Frozen)|| — Eat at least ___ servings|| (serving sizes listed are raw vegetables. Cooked vegetables equal ½ cup.)	
45 calorie serving	Serving size	75 calorie serving	Serving size	70 calorie serving	Serving size	40 calorie serving	Serving size	20 calorie serving	Serving size
Alcohol		Cottage		**Preferred foods**		**Occasional foods§**		**Preferred foods**	
Beer		(non-creamed)	½ c	Cereal dry, whole grain		Dried fruit		Water chestnuts	4
Regular	3½ oz	(creamed)	⅓ c	Bran flakes	⅔ c	Apricots	2	Zucchini	⅔ c
"Lite"	5 oz	Ricotta		Raisin bran	⅓ c	Dates	1½		
Liquor	⅔ oz	(part skim)	¼ c	Shredded wheat	½ c	Figs	1	**Occasional foods§**	
Wine		Milk		Crackers, whole grain	(see labels)	Prunes	1½		
Coolers	2½ oz	Skim, nonfat	1 c	Whole grain crisp bread	(see labels)	Raisins	2 T	Canned vegetables	½ c
Dry	1 oz	Buttermilk	1 c			Fruit juice		Pickle, sour	1 lg
Sweet	1 oz					Apple	⅓ c	Sauerkraut	⅔ c
						Cranberry	¼ c	Tomato juice	3 oz
								V-8 juice	4 oz

Evaporated diluted 1:2	1 c
Milk powder	1/3 c
Low fat, 1-2%	2/3 c
Whole	1/2 c
Buttermilk	1/2 c
Evaporated diluted 1:2	1/2 c
Yogurt, low-fat, plain	2/3 c
Egg	1

Pita pouches, whole grain	1/2 round
Popcorn, plain	3 c
Occasional foods§	
Bagel	1/2
Biscuit or muffin	1/2
Bread, white	1 sl
Cornbread (count 1 fat)	2" cubes
Cereal, dry, other, non-sugared	(see label)
Cereal, cooked, white	1/2 c
Crackers	
Graham (3)	2½" sq
Oat	7
Oyster	20
Saltines	6
Soda	5
Pasta, cooked	1/2 c
Pretzel sticks	25
Rice, cooked white	1/3 c
Roll, dinner	1 sm

Frozen fruit juice bar, (unsweetened)	1
Grapefruit	1/2 c
Orange	1/3 c
Pineapple	1/3 c
Prune	1/4 c

Reprinted with permission of The University of Alabama at Birmingham, c. 1990.

*The spectrum of energy densities of food groups in the EatRight program. Food groups to the right are lowest in energy density; highest in bulk, and require a longer time to eat.

†Weigh portions after cooking.

‡Cooked starches should represent at least half the total intake of starch.

§Up to two items per week.

‖The number of servings to be eaten in each category depends upon the caloric level of the diet prescribed. As commonly used examples: 4 vegetables, 4 fruits, 4 starch, 5 milk/meat, 3 fat servings per day is approximately 1030 kcal/day.

Table 2-2B   Foods that are 100 calories (or less) and contain 2 grams (or less) fat*

5 pieces hard candy	1 large date-filled oatmeal cookie
1 Fudgesicle	1 piece angel food cake ($\frac{1}{15}$ of
1 Popsicle	cake)
$\frac{1}{2}$ cup ice milk	6 gingersnaps
$\frac{1}{2}$ cup (4 oz) lowfat frozen yogurt	4 social tea cookies
$\frac{1}{2}$ cup gelatin dessert	12 animal crackers
1 large apple-filled oatmeal cookie	3 iced animal crackers

*For others, read labels. (Limit: 200 calories per week.)
Reprinted with permission of The University of Alabama at Birmingham, c. 1990.

In *Exchange Lists for Meal Planning*, developed by the American Diabetes Association and the American Dietetic Association, foods that have similar compositions of carbohydrate, protein, and fat are combined into one of six food groups, from which a variety of selections may be made (see Table 2-3). Varied calorie levels may be adapted by increasing or decreasing the servings from the different groups (see Table 2-4).

The diet also may consist of unlimited use of complex carbohydrates such as vegetables. It has been demonstrated that a high-fiber diet helps to improve blood-glucose control after a meal. The intake of saturated fat and cholesterol should be limited because of predisposition of the diabetic patient to hyperlipidemia and atherosclerotic vascular disease. Thus, fish, chicken, and low-fat dairy products are the preferred protein sources. Ingestion of simple sugars such as candy and sweetened carbonated beverages should be minimized to avoid hyperglycemic peaks.

Challenging the exchange system of meal planning is the use of a glycemic index, a measure of how much a given carbohydrate food will raise a person's blood sugar. Foods, such as white bread and white potatoes, that have a high glycemic index are expected to increase blood sugar most dramatically. However, many factors influence the body's response to a particular food, including the amount and type of fat and fiber in the meal; the timing, dosage, and type of medicines used; and function of the digestive tract. Research continues, but findings are still incomplete and inconclusive on the advantages of this index. For now, the exchange system of meal planning will remain the primary tool in planning snacks and meals.

Type I diabetic patients require an outside source of insulin because the body is unable to produce it. The type, dosage, and administration schedule depend on the patient's stage of growth, activity or exercise patterns, and eating habits. If the diabetic patient receives too much or too little insulin, hypoglycemia or hyperglycemia and diabetic ketoacidosis may occur.

Hypoglycemia also may result from excessive physical activity, irregular meal patterns, or inadequate food intake. In this case, a readily absorbed form of carbohydrate such as fruit juice, hard candy, sugar, or glucose solution should be taken immediately.

Table 2-3 Nutrition composition of the six diabetic exchange groups

Food group or Exchange	Serving size (example)	Carbohydrate (g)	Protein (g)	Fat (g)	Fat (kcal)
Fruits	1 medium apple	15	—	—	60
Vegetables	½ cup green beans	5	2	—	25
Starch	1 slice whole wheat bread	15	3	trace	80
Milk (skim)	8 oz	12	8	trace	90
Meat (medium-fat)	1 oz beef	—	7	5	75
Fat	1 tsp margarine	—	—	5	45

Table 2-4 Examples of dietary patterns using the diabetic exchange list*

	Numbers of exchanges per day	
	1200 kcal	1500 kcal
Fruit	3.0	4.0
Vegetable	4.0	4.0
Starch	4.0	5.5
Milk (skim)	2.0	2.0
Meat	3.5	5.0
Fat	4.5	5.0

*Example of 1200 and 1500-kcal diets made up of 50% carbohydrate, 20% protein, and 30% fat.

Hyperglycemia can result from stress, infection, overeating, or ingesting large amounts of concentrated sweets. Treatment may entail administration of rapid-acting insulin and if necessary correction of fluid and electrolyte imbalances by using intravenous fluids. Activity and exercise tend to reduce the need for insulin, since exercise lowers blood-glucose levels. The diabetic should be advised that he or she needs 10 to 15 g of carbohydrate/hour of moderate exercise and 20 to 30 g/hour of vigorous exercise.

Type II diabetic patients are relatively insulin-resistant because of excessive adiposity. The cornerstone of dietary therapy involves weight reduction. Exchange lists are useful in planning menus for patients with either type I or II diabetes.

Dietary management of diabetes has changed dramatically over the past few decades as we have progressed from the high-fat, carbohydrate-restricted diets to low-fat, high complex-carbohydrate diets, and now the controversial glycemic index approach, which even includes sugars in the diet. However, until our understanding improves, it is recommended that diabetic patients continue to curtail the use of fat, sugar, salt, and alcohol and to increase their intake of complex carbohydrates and foods high in fiber. The diabetic exchange lists implement these recommendations and allow for individual differences and long-term management of diabetes.

DIET, HYPERLIPIDEMIA, AND CORONARY ARTERY DISEASE

Coronary artery disease (CAD) and its clinical presentation—angina, heart attack, and sudden death—represent a public health problem of enormous magnitude. CAD is responsible for more than 500,000 deaths in the United States each year, more than all other diseases combined, including all forms of cancer. Although elevated serum cholesterol is the major predictive risk factor of CAD (Fig. 2-3 and Table 2-5), the disease is clearly multifactorial and life-style related. Modifiable factors in addition to serum cholesterol include hyperlipidemia, cigarette smoking, diabetes mellitus, severe obesity, and hypertension. Fixed risk factors include family history, age, and male sex. A major modifiable risk factor is hypercholesterolemia, which in approximately 99% of cases is not hereditary but life-style related, particularly to diet. Figures 2-4A–C show manifestations of various types hyperlipidemia.

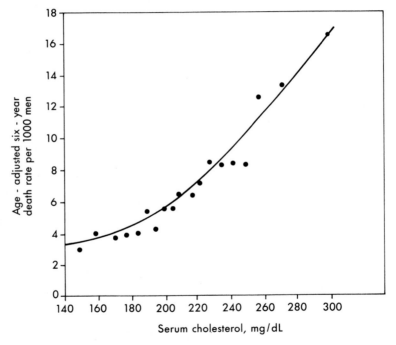

Fig. 2-3 The relationship of serum cholesterol to coronary heart disease (CHD) death in 361,662 men 35 to 57 years of age during an average follow-up of six years. Each point represents median value for 5% of the population. Key points are as follows: (1) risk increases steadily, particularly above levels of 200 mg/dl; and (2) the magnitude of the increased risk is large, fourfold in the top 10% as compared with the bottom 10%. (From NIH Report of the National Cholesterol Education Program Expert Panel on Detection, Evaluation, and Treatment of High Blood Cholesterol in Adults. *Arch Intern Med*, Jan-Mar 1988, 148:36-69.)

Table 2-5 Plasma lipid concentrations and association with coronary artery disease (CAD) according to percentiles of lipid distribution*

Age (yr)	CAD risk: percentile:	Total cholesterol (mg/dl)			HDL cholesterol (mg/dl)			Triglycerides (mg/dl)	
		Normal 50	Moderate 75	High 90	Increased 5	Normal 50	Decreased 95	50†	95†
Men									
5-19		155	170	185	35	55	75	58	111
20-24		165	185	205	30	45	65	78	165
25-29		180	200	225	30	45	65	88	204
30-34		190	215	240	30	45	60	102	253
35-39		200	225	250	30	45	60	109	316
40-44		205	230	250	25	45	65	123	318
45-69		215	235	260	30	50	70	117	261
70+		205	230	250	30	50	75	115	239
Women									
5-19		160	175	190	35	55	70	68	120
20-24		170	190	215	35	55	80	80	168
25-34		175	195	220	35	55	80	75	161
35-39		185	205	230	35	55	80	83	205
40-44		195	215	235	35	60	90	68	191
45-49		205	225	250	35	60	85	94	223
50-54		220	240	265	35	60	90	103	223
55+		230	250	275	35	60	95	111	271

*Adapted from the Lipid Research Clinics Population Studies Data. Book: I. The Prevalence. Study publication 80-1527. Bethesda, MD, NIH, 1980.
†An independent relationship to coronary artery disease has not been established for triglycerides.

Cholesterol and triglycerides are transported in circulation with phospholipids and apoproteins as water-soluble lipoproteins. There are five major classes of lipoproteins. Chylomicrons, formed in the intestine from dietary fat and mainly composed of triglycerides, are normally cleared from circulation within four hours after a meal. Very low–density lipoproteins (VLDL) are synthesized by the liver and transport triglycerides even in the fasting state. Intermediate-density lipoproteins (IDL) contain approximately equal amounts of cholesterol and triglyceride, are formed from VLDL, and are normally quickly removed from the blood or further degraded to LDL. Low-density lipoproteins (LDL) are the major carriers of cholesterol and normally account for about 50% to 70% of total blood cholesterol. Along with their apolipoprotein B component, LDL are the most atherogenic lipid particles. The presence of a second large protein, apolipoprotein (a), appears to increase further the atherogenicity of this particle. High-density lipoproteins (HDL) appear to transport cholesterol from peripheral tissues to the liver, and whether by this or other mechanisms are associated with a reduced risk of CAD.

The diet-heart hypothesis holds that diet affects lipid and lipoprotein levels, which in turn can alter risk of CAD. The following sections discuss the validity of this hypothesis.

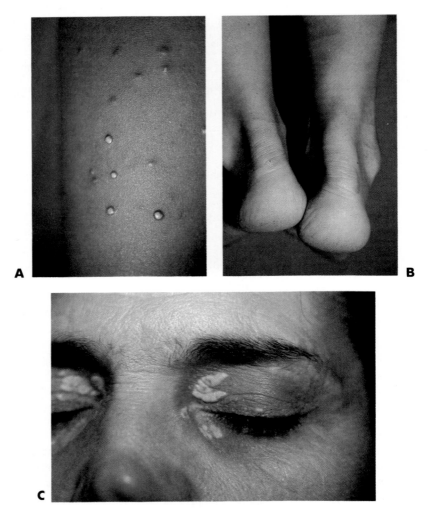

Fig. 2-4 **A**, Eruptive xanthomas of types I and V hyperlipidemia. **B**, Thickening of Achille's tendons in Type II familial hyperlipidemia. **C**, Xanthelasma of the eyelids in type II hyperlipidemia.

Diet and lipid levels

The effect of diet on serum lipid levels has been proved beyond any reasonable doubt.

Saturated fat has the most profound cholesterol-raising effect. All animal fats except those in fish and shellfish are highly saturated and therefore are firm at room temperature. Sources are whole milk, ice cream, butter, cheese, and red meat.

Polyunsaturated fats depress plasma cholesterol, and ω-3 fatty acids found primarily in fish oil lower triglyceride levels and, to a minor extent, blood cholesterol. Polyunsaturated fat is derived from plant and seafood oils and is liquid at room temperature. Exceptions are coconut oil, cocoa butter (from chocolate), and palm oil, all of which are saturated cholesterol-raising vegetable oils often used in commercial products because they provide for a longer shelf life. Commercial margarines and shortenings are hydrogenated (hardened) to variable extents, which can reduce their cholesterol-lowering ability. Gram for gram, saturated fat is up to two times more cholesterol-elevating than polyunsaturated fat is cholesterol-lowering.

Despite the advantage of unsaturated fat over saturated fat, complex carbohydrates are a preferred dietary substitute. Reasons for avoiding larger intake of even unsaturated fats include the following: 1) the high caloric density of the oils and margarines, 2) the increased risk of cholesterol gallstones, 3) increased cholesterol synthesis in some hypertriglyceridemic patients, and 4) unknown long-term consequences of large intakes of polyunsaturated fats. Fish, which is a source of lipid-lowering ω-3 fatty acids, is recommended as a substitute for meat; however, the use of fish oil supplements has not been recommended pending more data on their safety and effectiveness.

Monounsaturated fats, found mainly in peanut and olive oils, are preferable to saturated fats and may have a cholesterol-lowering effect according to some studies. Most reports, however, have shown no independent effects of monounsaturated fats on cholesterol levels.

Dietary cholesterol is poorly absorbed (about 40%) and tends to cause inhibition of cholesterol synthesis. Nevertheless, the net effect of increased intake is elevation of plasma cholesterol. Average intake in the United States is approximately 400 mg/day, with about half coming from egg yolk and foods processed with egg yolk and the other half from meat, fish, poultry, and dairy products.

Complex carbohydrates such as unrefined starches in bread and cereal products, fruits, and vegetables, in contrast to refined sugars, tend to have a triglyceride-lowering effect. However, there is no consistent effect of dietary fiber; some fibers, such as pectin, oat bran, and guargum favorably effect cholesterol levels, whereas wheat bran generally has no effect.

Alcohol consumption tends to raise levels of triglycerides and HDL cholesterol, particularly the HDL-3 subfraction.

Lipids and coronary artery disease

Elevated total plasma cholesterol is a strong predictor of risk for CAD, particularly in young adult men. Most of the plasma cholesterol is carried in low-density lipoprotein (LDL), which is itself directly correlated with risk of CAD. The risk of heart disease increases more rapidly at higher cholesterol levels: about twofold when total cholesterol rises from 200 to 250 mg/dl and over threefold when the cholesterol level rises from 200 to 300 mg/dl (see Fig. 2-3).

In populations with high risk of CAD, low plasma HDL cholesterol appears to be a significant predictor of CAD. On the other hand, in populations with low CAD risk and with low LDL concentrations, HDL levels are also frequently low. Thus, low HDL is of particular concern for risk of CAD in populations where LDL levels are high.

Most studies have not demonstrated an independent association between triglyceride levels and CAD, although triglyceride abnormalities may accompany or reflect other lipid disturbances that do accelerate atherosclerosis.

Normal lipid levels

Table 2-5 shows the distribution of total and HDL cholesterol and triglyceride levels in men, women, and children and relative risks of CAD. On the basis of worldwide epidemiologic data, the upper limit of the desirable range for total plasma cholesterol is about 200 mg/dl. People with moderate and high-risk cholesterol levels (>75th percentile) should be treated first with diet, with the goal being a level of less than 240 mg/dl (LDL cholesterol <160 mg/dl) for adults without CAD and fewer than two risk factors, and less than 200 mg/dl (LDL <130 mg/dl) in the presence of CAD or two or more risk factors. Ideally, total plasma cholesterol should be between about 100 and 190 mg/dl. A combination of diet and medication may be necessary in patients who do not respond to dietary therapy.

The upper limit of normal for plasma triglycerides is not well defined but is currently considered as the 95th percentile, or about 250 mg/dl for most adults.

Dietary treatment and prevention of coronary artery disease

Recent large-scale clinical trials have clearly demonstrated that reduction in total blood cholesterol favorably alters the risk of development of CAD and the progression of established disease. Data from the Lipid Research Clinics Coronary Primary Prevention Trial suggest that for every 1% decrease in cholesterol, a 2% reduction in the risk of CAD can be expected. There seems to be little doubt that appropriate dietary changes will afford significant protection against CAD. For this reason, the following general recommendations, similar to those of the American Heart Association and the Inter-Society Commission for Heart Disease Resources, have been made by the National Institutes of Health (NIH) Consensus Development Panel and National Cholesterol Education Program:

1. People with high-risk cholesterol levels (>90th percentile, Table 2-5) should have diet modifications according to the guidelines for type II hyperlipoproteinemia (Table 2-6). These dietary recommendations are generally suitable for hypercholesterolemic children and other family members. Drugs should be added only if the response is inadequate.
2. Adults with moderate-risk cholesterol levels (between 75th and 90th percentiles) should follow the dietary guidelines above, but very few should require drug therapy.
3. For all Americans older than 2 years of age, dietary changes to reduce total fat to 30% of calories from the current level of about 40% should be encouraged; saturated fat should be reduced to less than 10% of calories, polyunsaturated fat should be increased but to no more than 10%, and daily cholesterol intake should be reduced to 300 mg or less.

Table 2-6   Dietary guidelines for hyperlipoproteinemia

	Type I	Type IIA, IIB, III	Type IV	Type V
Calories	For ideal weight	For ideal weight	For ideal weight	For ideal weight
Fat	<20% of kcal	reduce stepwise to <30% and to <25% of calories as needed; reduce saturated fat to <10% and to <7% as needed	same as IIA	<20%
Cholesterol	Not restricted	Reduce stepwise to <300 and to <200 mg/day as needed	<300 mg/day	<300 mg/day
Carbohydrate	Not limited	At least 50% of calories, primarily as vegetables, fruits, and unrefined starches	Same as IIA	Same as IIA
Alcohol	Avoid	<1 oz/day	<1 oz/day	Avoid

Classification of abnormal lipoprotein patterns

An abnormal lipoprotein pattern is not necessarily a disease entity. When elevated blood lipid levels are identified, there are four categories of causation to consider:
1. A spurious value—e.g., hyperchylomicronemia found in a nonfasting state.
2. A genetic disorder, identified by its pattern of inheritance.
3. A dietary-induced disorder—that is, primarily reflecting dietary indiscretions.
4. A secondary disorder—that is, a result of an underlying disease or use of certain drugs.

In considering the patterns of hyperlipoproteinemia, it is useful from a practical standpoint to recall that types I, III, and V are relatively uncommon and that types II and IV are quite common. Thus, hypercholesterolemia usually reflects a type II pattern (increased LDL), and hypertriglyceridemia usually reflects a type IV pattern (increased VLDL). Table 2-7 outlines the typical features and secondary causes of the hyperlipoproteinemias. See Figure 2-4A–C for examples of clinical manifestations of some of these lipid abnormalities.

Lipid screening

All adults, when first seen and at no more than 5-year intervals, should have total plasma cholesterol and triglycerides measured using a fasting sample. Elevated lipid levels should be confirmed by at least two determinations, one of which should include lipoprotein fractionation. If total cholesterol or triglycerides

Table 2-7 Typical features and secondary causes of hyperlipidemia

Type	Plasma	Laboratory features*			Clinical signs	Secondary causes
		Lipoproteins	Cholesterol	Triglycerides		
I	Clear plasma, cream layer	↑ Chylomicrons	↑	↑↑ - ↑↑↑ (often >2000)	Abdominal pain after fat intake, pancreatitis, hepatosplenomegaly, eruptive xanthomas, lipemia retinalis	Pancreatitis, insulinopenic diabetes, dysproteinemia
IIA	Clear	↑ LDL	↑ - ↑↑	Normal	Tendon, planar, tuberous xanthomas, xanthelasma, corneal arcus, vascular disease	Hypothyroidism, Cushing's obstructive liver disease, nephrotic syndrome, dysproteinemia, porphyria; thiazides, beta-adrenergic blockers, estrogen, oral contraceptives, pregnancy
IIB	Clear or turbid	↑ VLDL				

III	Clear or turbid; often cream layer	↑ IDL	↑	↑	Palmar, tuberous xanthomas, corneal arcus, vascular disease; obesity often present	Diabetes, hypothyroidism, dysproteinemia
IV	Often turbid	↑ VLDL	Normal or ↑	↑ - ↑ ↑ (usually <1000)	Eruptive xanthomas (if triglycerides are ↑ ↑)	Diabetes, nephrotic syndrome, renal dialysis, glycogen storage disease, dysproteinemia; thiazides, beta-adrenergic blockers, estrogens, oral contraceptives, pregnancy
V	Cream layer, turbid plasma	↑ Chylomicrons ↑ VLDL	↑ - ↑ ↑	↑ ↑ ↑ - ↑ ↑ ↑ (often >2000)	Abdominal pain after fat intake, pancreatitis, hepatosplenomegaly, eruptive xanthomas, lipemia retinalis	Insulinopenic diabetes, pancreatitis, dysproteinemia

*Sample drawn after overnight fast. Plasma characteristics are seen after plasma sample has set overnight in a refrigerator. Arrows indicate direction and extent of lipid change.

↑ = mildly increased; ↑ ↑ = significantly increased.

are above the 90th to 95th percentile (see Table 2-5) and they are not the result of another disease, other family members should be screened for genetic forms of hyperlipidemia. Children with lipid disorders probably should be identified by a carefully obtained family history of premature (before 60 years of age) heart disease rather than by routine blood screening.

In most cases, the pattern of hyperlipoproteinemia can be diagnosed on the basis of the level of total cholesterol and triglycerides and perhaps visual inspection of plasma stored overnight at 4° C (see Table 2-7). If the triglyceride level is less than 800 mg/dl, LDL cholesterol can be reasonably estimated using the following formula:

LDL chol = total chol-(triglycerides/5 + HDL chol) . . . where HDL chol can be estimated at 45 mg/dl if unknown.

An LDL cholesterol value greater than 160 mg/dl is suggestive of a type IIA or IIB pattern, whereas if triglycerides are elevated and LDL cholesterol is less than 160 mg/dl, it suggests a type IV pattern. Classification of risk for CAD is based on the presence of a type II pattern according to the following:

LDL levels

Below 130 mg/dl   desirable level
130-159 mg/dl   borderline risk
160 mg/dl or above   high risk

Once a lipoprotein abnormality is confirmed, any medications that may be causing the hyperlipidemia should be stopped if medically possible (see Table 2-7), and the lipid level should be reevaluated. If the lipid level is still elevated, secondary causes should be ruled out.

HYPERTENSION

Even by conservative standards, it is estimated that 20% of the American population is hypertensive. In the vast majority of these individuals, there is no simple explanation and no known cause. Since the late 1960s, mortality rates for cardiovascular disease have drastically declined, partly because of the introduction and general use of antihypertensive medications. There is, however, strong evidence that diet can play a major role in the prevention and management of hypertension.

Sodium and potassium

Sodium is present in varying amounts in all foods and is a common additive in many prepared and processed foods. As an essential nutrient, the estimated minimum requirement for infants, children, and adults ranges from 100 to 200 mg per day. Average sodium intake in the American population is about 20 times that requirement, or about 4000 to 5000 mg/day.

In general, populations such as the United States with a very high sodium intake have a very high prevalence of hypertension. In fact, clinical trials have shown that modest sodium restriction is effective in lowering blood pressure in certain people and that it improves the action of diuretics in lowering blood pressure. But response is not uniform, and there is at present no easy way to identify the patients who are more sensitive to sodium.

Since there is no known benefit from consuming sodium in an amount beyond that needed to meet daily losses, and since there is evidence of risk associated with diets high in sodium content, moderate reductions in sodium intake are recommended. An intake of 2000 to 3000 mg per day is achievable and considered palatable after a brief period of adaptation. Because most canned, frozen, and prepared convenience foods contain hidden amounts of salt, reduction of sodium intake requires careful attention to the selection of these foods as well as reducing the amount of added salt.

Tables 2-8A and B provide a general guideline for several levels of sodium restriction.

In contrast to sodium, diets high in potassium seem to have a favorable effect on blood pressure. A liberal intake of foods rich in potassium may partially offset the blood pressure–raising effects of sodium. The usual adult intake ranges from 2000 to 6000 mg/day, and it appears that intake on the upper end of the range is optimal.

Table 2-8A   Modified diets—sodium

Daily sodium (Na) intake*	Food limitations	Practicality
5 to 6 g Na (= 12.5 to 15 g salt)	Includes table salt, heavily or visibly salted items	Average American diet
4 g Na (= 10 g salt)	No additional salt on tray or at table	Practical for home use
3 g Na (= 7.5 g salt)	Food only lightly salted in preparation; restrict heavily or visibly salted items (potato chips, pretzels, crackers, pickles, olives, relishes, sauces, most soups); no salt on tray	Practical for home use
2 g Na (= 5 g salt)	Above limitations plus no salt in food preparation; avoid most processed foods (canned foods, dry cereals, luncheon meats, bacon, ham, cheese) unless calculated into diet; regular bread, butter, milk in limited amounts	Fairly practical for home use with cooperative patient
1 g Na (= 2.5 g salt)	Above limitations plus use of only salt-free bread	Practical for home use with only unusually cooperative patient
0.5 g Na (= 1.25 g salt)	Above limitations plus limitation of meat (4 oz/day), eggs, some vegetables; milk (1 pt/day) and salt-free butter allowed	Not practical for home use

*1 g Na = 43 mEq; 1 mEq Na = 23 mg; 1 g NaCl = 2.5 g Na; 1 g Na = 0.4 g NaCl.

Table 2-8B   High-sodium foods to omit on a sodium-restricted diet

CONDIMENTS:

Pickles, olives, relishes, salted nuts, meat tenderizers, commercial salad dressings, monosodium glutamate (Accent®), steak sauce, ketchup, soy sauce, Worchestershire sauce, horseradish sauce, chili sauce, commercial mustard, onion salt, garlic salt, celery salt, butter salt, seasoned salt

BREADS:

Salted crackers

MEAT, FISH, POULTRY, CHEESE, AND SUBSTITUTES:

Cured, smoked, and processed meats such as ham, bacon, corned beef, chipped beef, weiners, luncheon meats, bologna, salt pork, regular canned salmon and tuna; all cheese except low sodium and cottage cheese; TV dinners, pizza, frozen Italian entrees, imitation sausage and bacon

BEVERAGES:

Commercial buttermilk, instant hot cocoa mixes

SOUPS:

Commercial canned and dehydrated soups (except low-sodium soups), bouillon, consommé

VEGETABLES:

Sauerkraut, hominy, pork and beans, canned tomato and vegetable juices

FATS:

Gravy, regular peanut butter

POTATO OR POTATO SUBSTITUTES:

Potato chips, corn chips, salted popcorn, pretzels, frozen potato casseroles, commercially packaged rice and noodle mixes, dehydrated potatoes and potato mixes, bread stuffing

Obesity and hypertension

As a group, hypertensive patients tend to be overweight. There is a small but statistically significant association between blood pressure and body weight. However, the majority of obese people are not hypertensive. Careful statistical analyses of the association have indicated that the apparent association between obesity and hypertension is largely explained by increased age, greater lean body mass, and the broad body build that is associated with increased weight rather than by body fatness per se.

Not surprisingly, weight reduction seems to be effective in reducing the blood pressure of certain hypertensive patients. The mechanism underlying the well-established hypotensive effect of weight reduction is still unexplained but at least in part is related to changes in dietary factors rather than loss of body fat itself. For most overweight people with mild hypertension, the option of a well-balanced program of weight control carries little risk and at least some temporary benefit in lowering blood pressure. A concerted effort to modify diet—reduce energy intake to achieve and maintain ideal weight, decrease sodium intake, and increase potassium intake—should be considered before resorting to drug therapy.

Dietary fat and calcium

A diet relatively low in fat, and one in which most fat is polyunsaturated, seems to promote a lower blood pressure than do high-fat diets with a preponderance of saturated fat. Fat intake should be limited to 25% to 30% of the total calories, and intake of saturated fat should be minimized.

The mechanisms by which calcium affects blood pressure are poorly defined. A number of studies have shown that low levels of calcium intake tend to be associated with increased levels of blood pressure. However, results of intervention trials have been inconclusive or conflicting. It appears that only certain population subgroups may be responsive to the blood pressure–lowering effects of calcium.

A word about prevention: Although the specific causes of hypertension may not be known, we do know that once initiated, hypertension may be self-sustaining. When cardiovascular damage has occurred, even removal of the causative agent may be ineffective in reducing blood pressure to normal levels. This accents the importance of modifying diet as a preventive measure.

DIET AND CANCER

The link between diet and cancer has received much attention in recent years. Although a large number of nutrients have been implicated in modifying the development of malignancies, much is still unknown about the specific relationship between what we eat and our risk of cancer. Because cancer is the second leading cause of death in the United States, and because surviving the deadliest forms—colon, breast, and lung—has not yet substantially increased, prevention through diet as well as through other means could have a major impact on the American population.

Research has not yet conclusively proved the causal effect of any specific nutrient in cancer development. Those thought to play a role, either in the development or prevention of cancer, include the following:

High dietary fat. This has been strongly implicated to increase risk for several cancers, including breast, colon, prostate, and ovarian malignancies. Red meat intake has particularly been associated with risk for colon cancer. Obesity has been linked epidemiologically with increased rates of cancers of various organs, especially of the endometrium, and breast. The associations with endometrial and breast cancers are probably not because of caloric excess but are more likely due to changes in circulating estrogens in obese women.

Dietary fiber. This has received a great deal of publicity because of its possible role in protecting against colon cancer. Certain types of insoluble fiber found in whole-grain foods, such as cellulose, hemicellulose, and lignins, appear to have a protective effect against colon cancer; but some of the apparent effects of fiber noted in epidemiologic studies may actually be a reflection of other factors, such as reduced fat intake.

Vitamin A. Vitamin A and its related retinoid compounds provide some of the more firmly established diet-cancer links. Clinical trials in humans appear to show that retinoids are protective against premalignant lesions of the lung and buccal mucosa. Their effects on other organs, such as the breast, oropharynx, and skin, are being studied; because of the risk of toxicity, supplementation is not recommended.

Folic acid. Folate status correlates inversely with the presence of cervical dysplasia in women with human papilloma virus infection and with atypical bronchial metaplasia in cigarette smokers.

Vitamin C. Evidence of the preventive effects of vitamin C on human cancer is weak. Studies showing lower rates of gastric, esophageal, and laryngeal cancers in people with high vitamin C intakes may be confounded by its presence in foods containing other possibly protective compounds.

Vitamin E. Vitamin E has more popular support than scientific data behind its role in cancer prevention. Its ability to protect lipid membranes against oxidation suggests that vitamin E may play a role in inhibiting the action of carcinogens.

Selenium. Also an antioxidant, selenium may have a protective effect particularly against cancers of the gastrointestinal tract. However, because the selenium content of food is largely dependent on the selenium content of the soil, and because the safe range of supplementation is narrow, dietary changes are not recommended.

Alcohol. This is not itself a carcinogen but promotes cancer development in several organs. Excessive alcohol consumption is the major cause of hepatic cirrhosis in the United States, and the incidence of liver cancer is greatly increased in people with cirrhosis. Excess alcohol also interacts with cigarette smoking to increase risk of oral, pharyngeal, and esophageal cancer. Even moderate alcohol intake appears to increase the risk for breast cancer.

Dietary recommendations for cancer prevention

The National Cancer Institute, the National Research Council, and the American Cancer Society have issued reasonable dietary guidelines for cancer prevention based on current information. They include the following:

- Avoid obesity.
- Decrease total fat intake to 30% or less of total calories.
- Increase intake of whole-grain foods.
- Increase intake of dark green, deep yellow, and orange vegetables.
- Eat salt-cured, smoked, and nitrite-cured foods in moderation.
- If alcohol is used, it should be used in moderation.

At this time, the use of nutritional supplements for cancer prevention is not recommended because most of the desired effects are presumed to be achievable through a prudent diet.

NUTRITION AND ORAL HEALTH

Diet, oral health, and total-body nutritional status are closely intertwined. Because the mouth is the entry point for nutrients, total-body nutritional status is dependent on the integrity of dental tissue and oral soft tissue. The converse also is true, because abnormal oral tissue often occurs as a result of nutrient imbalances. Finally, the diet also influences oral health through local stimulation of the cariogenic flora in dental plaque adhering to teeth.

A lack of nutrients during critical periods of growth exert profound effects on the chemical composition of teeth, the time of eruption, and the development of the salivary glands.

Fluoride is a beneficial element in food and water affecting oral health. Classical epidemiological studies established the inverse relationship between decayed, missing, and filled teeth (DMFT), and fluoride concentration in the water supply. Ingested fluoride becomes incorporated into the hydroxyapatite structure of the developing tooth enamel and exerts its anticaries activity by increasing the enamel's resistance to acid solubility, aiding in the remineralization of demineralized enamel, and by exerting an antibacterial effect when given in high topical concentrations.

Use of fluoride supplements beginning at an early age enhances the formation of caries-resistant teeth. The level of recommended water fluoridation is approximately 1 ppm, but may be less depending on latitude and other environmental factors. This level of supplementation will provide approximately 1 mg of fluoride/day to the average adult who drinks a liter of water. Infants not receiving fluoride from other sources should receive 0.25 mg/day. From ages 2 to 3 years, 0.5 mg/day is recommended, whereas from ages 3 to 14 years, 1 mg/day is recommended. Fluoride also may be given through topical therapy and oral lozenges. Care should be exercised not to exceed optimal doses of fluoride from the water and other food and toothpaste sources to avoid the problem of fluorosis (mottling).

The effect of nutrients on oral health

Other nutrients also affect the integrity of soft tissue, salivary composition, pulp circulation, and dentin metabolism, and they may have a direct effect on healing and repairing mechanisms in the periodontium. Vitamin C deficiency is a graphic example of this influence.

Figure 2-5 shows the easily bleeding gums as well as loosening and loss of teeth in scurvy. These findings may reflect vitamin C-induced defects in oral epithelial basement membrane and periodontal collagen fiber synthesis.

Dental caries and carbohydrates

Dental caries is one of the most rampant public health problems in the United States. Fermentable carbohydrates in the diet of individuals with poor oral hygiene and lack of fluoride have been implicated in the development of tooth decay, but the link between carbohydrates and caries is complex, because of the various factors entering in the etiology of this disease.

Several well-controlled clinical trials have confirmed the role of sugar in tooth decay. However, those and succeeding studies also have implicated tooth integrity, frequency and type of carbohydrates eaten, stickiness of food, bacterial plaque characteristics, and flow and composition of saliva as contributing factors. Therefore, dental caries is a complex, multifactorial disease, and prevention must attack many components. Dietary guidelines have consistently recommended

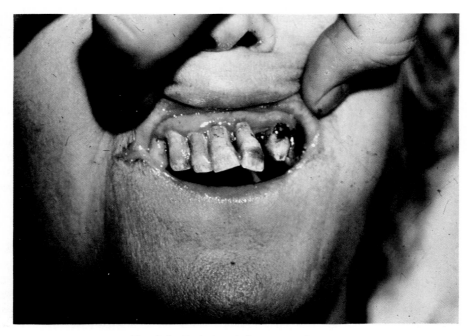

Fig. 2-5   Periodontal disease seen in scurvy.

eating a balanced diet that limits between-meal snacking and sugar-containing foods.

In summary, oral health is a reflection of total-body nutritional status and is affected both before and after eruption by nutrient intake. This effect persists throughout life. Future research will further delineate mechanisms and optional conditions for the prevention of oral disease.

OSTEOPOROSIS

Osteoporosis is defined as a loss of bone mass with an increased tendency for fractures to occur with minimal stress or trauma. This definition provides a useful conceptual framework, but it does have limitations. For example, patients with low bone mass may never have a fracture, and conversely, fractures may occur in the absence of reduced bone mass. In addition, osteoporotic patients may differ in numerous respects such as histologic appearance of the bone; rates and patterns of bone synthesis and resorption; rates of calcium absorption; and serum concentrations of parathyroid hormone, vitamin D, and calcitonin. Thus, the many factors leading to the development of osteoporosis and to its clinical presentation are still being studied.

Fractures due to osteoporosis are responsible for significant disability, morbidity, mortality, and expense (an estimated $6 billion in health care expenditures each year). Approximately 1.2 million fractures due to osteoporosis occur each year in the United States, and they primarily involve the vertebrae, hip, and distal forearm. The hip fracture is the most dangerous and is associated with a 12% to 20% increase in death rate within 12 months of the fracture in women.

Factors contributing to bone mass

A number of factors enter into the equation for the production and maintenance of healthy bones.

Age. Bone mass increases until approximately 30 years of age. After a period of stabilization, the phenomenon of age-associated bone loss begins for both men and women. This is especially true for women during approximately the first 10 years of the postmenopausal period, when a substantial reduction in bone mass occurs concomitantly with a reduction in estrogen production. By about the fifth decade, this age-associated bone loss begins to affect men and becomes progressively more significant through the remaining life span for both men and women. However, the rate of bone loss may be reduced by changes in some of the factors discussed below.

The greater the amount of absolute bone mass attained by age 30, the greater the amount of bone available in reserve to offset the age-associated bone loss and therefore protect against future fracture occurrences. Thus, a person who has a low bone mass by 30 years of age has an increased risk for early osteoporotic fractures.

Heredity and body size. The quantity and quality of absolute bone mass attained by maturity is associated with numerous inherited factors. Factors associated with reduced bone mass include female gender, Caucasian or Asiatic descent, small stature, leanness, family history of osteoporosis, and long-term lactose intolerance. Conversely, factors associated with a greater bone mass include the counterparts to the above: male, black, large stature, and obesity.

Nutrition. The integrity of bone mass is related to calcium intake throughout life, especially during the 30-year period of bone mass accretion. The RDA for calcium is 1200 mg for ages 11 to 24 years and 800 mg for the years thereafter. Unfortunately, studies have shown that calcium intake is substantially below the RDA for virtually all age categories in both men and women.

Excessive protein intake enhances calcium excretion in the urine. Since excessive protein intake is common in Western culture, with intake often twice the RDA, there are concerns that this dietary pattern may result in a chronic negative calcium balance and loss of bone mass.

Phosphorus-rich foods may reduce the dietary calcium-to-phosphorus ratio and also disturb calcium balance. Soft drinks and processed meats are examples of foods high in phosphorus. In addition, increased sodium intake may lead to negative calcium balance by increasing urinary calcium excretion.

Other life-style factors. Use of alcohol, tobacco, and caffeine have a negative influence on bone mass as does a sedentary life-style. Exercise throughout the life cycle, especially weight-bearing exercise, is crucial in maintaining skeletal health, and is an important preventive measure to counteract age-associated bone loss.

Medical and/or surgical conditions or treatments. Several types of therapy, such as long-term use of glucocorticoids or anticonvulsants, and several conditions such as hyperparathyroidism, multiparity, resection of the stomach or small intestine, and thyrotoxicosis, have an adverse effect on calcium balance and bone mass.

Treatment

Because osteoporosis is usually multifactorial in origin, treatment remains controversial and investigational. The strategy for the prevention of fractures is to increase bone synthesis and/or reduce bone resorption. Several recommendations have been made by the National Institutes of Health 1984 Consensus Development Conference on Osteoporosis:
- Increase elemental calcium intake to 1000 to 1500 mg/day.
- Institute a program of modest weight-bearing exercise.
- Consider vitamin D supplementation in people at risk for vitamin D deficiency (for example, those receiving minimal exposure to sunlight or those with fat malabsorption).

Researchers continue to assess the indications for and effectiveness of other treatments, including calcitonin, fluoride, anabolic steroids, the 1-34 amino acid fragment of parathyroid hormone, vitamin D analogs, and diphosphonates.

Finally, there is unanimous agreement that the major thrust in the management of osteoporosis should be a program of prevention, especially before the age of attaining maximal bone mass. This approach should include regular weight-bearing exercise, avoidance of alcohol, tobacco, and caffeine, and a well-balanced diet including adequate intake of calcium and appropriate, not excessive, amounts of protein, sodium and phosphorus.

NUTRITIONAL ANEMIAS

Anemia, common to many types of nutritional deficiencies, can be defined as a lack of circulating red blood cells associated with the diminished oxygen-carrying capacity of the blood due to a lack of hemoglobin. Anemia is considered nutritional in origin when the intake of one or more essential nutrients is implicated in the etiology of the anemia. Table 2-9 identifies the causes of nutritional anemias based on cell size or mean corpuscular volume (MCV). Figures 2-6A and B show examples of microcytic (small) and macrocytic (large) cells. However, a relative nutrient deficiency may exist in the face of normal dietary intake if metabolic requirements are high (as for folic acid in hemolysis or pregnancy) or if external losses are great (as with loss of iron from chronic gastrointestinal bleeding).

Symptoms of anemia include early onset of fatigue with exertion as well as exercise intolerance, even to the point of cardiac or cerebral ischemia. This is especially true if vascular disease is present. Resting tachycardia with a pulse greater than 100 beats/min is a helpful diagnostic sign because it indicates the body's adaptation to the diminished oxygen-carrying capacity in the blood. Pallor of the mucous membranes (conjunctiva, buccal cavity, tongue) and skin may provide a clue to the presence of anemia, but unfortunately pallor does not correspond closely with the hematocrit.

Table 2-9   Causes of nutritional anemias by cell size

Microcytic (MCV <80)
  Fe
  Cu
  Vitamin B_6 (pyridoxine)

Normocytic (MCV 80-100)
  Protein-calorie malnutrition

Macrocytic (MCV >100)
  Vitamin B_{12}
  Folate

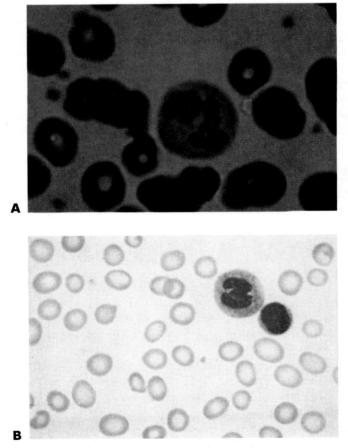

A

B

Fig. 2-6   **A,** Blood cells in macrocytic anemia; notice the hypersegmented polymor-phonuclear leukocytes. **B,** Blood cells in microcytic anemia.

It is important to remember that anemia almost never occurs as an isolated finding; a nutritional deficiency sufficient to limit the production of red blood cells usually affects other cells with a high turnover rate such as leukocytes, platelets, and enterocytes.

Most cases of megaloblastic anemia are accompanied by reddening and soreness of the tongue along with loss of lingual papillae. These changes make eating difficult and impose even further limitations on food choices.

Iron deficiency

Anemia due to lack of iron is the most common form of nutritional anemia and is perhaps the most common nutritional deficiency in the world. In men, iron equilibrium is accomplished by the absorption of 1 mg/day, on the average, from a diet containing the RDA of 10 mg of iron. This replaces the small amounts of iron lost by both men and women each day from minor injuries and shedding of epithelial cells. However, during their childbearing years, women also lose an average of 30 mg of elemental iron during each menstrual period, imposing a demand for an additional 0.5 mg, or a total of 1.5 mg per day, to maintain equilibrium. For premenopausal women, the RDA has been set at 15 mg/day.

A suspicion of iron deficiency anemia is supported by a low level of serum iron, usually less than 50 mg/dl, and an increase in the total iron-binding capacity (TIBC) greater than 400 mg/dl. Normally, TIBC is approximately one-third saturated; lower values are suggestive of iron deficiency. Table 2-10 presents some of the characteristic laboratory findings in iron deficiency.

It is always advisable to establish the cause of iron deficiency and to distinguish between inadequate nutritional intake and correctable causes of blood

Table 2-10 Laboratory findings in nutritional anemias

	Normal	Deficiency states		
		Iron	Folate	B$_{12}$
RBC morphology	Normocytic	Hypochromic, microcytic	Macrocytic (macroovalocytes)	Hyperchromic (macroovalocytes)
MCV μ^3	83-99	<80	>100	>100
MCHC %	32-36	<32	>32	
Hypersegmented neutrophils	Absent	Absent	Present	Present
Bone marrow	Normal	Normoblastic	Megaloblastic	Megaloblastic
Stainable iron in marrow	Normal	Absent	Normal or high	Normal or high
Serum iron, μg/ml	0.50-1.50	<.50	>1.50	>1.50
TIBC mg/ml	2.70-4.00	>4.00	>4.00	Normal or high
Serum ferritin ng/ml	10-300	<10	Normal or high	Normal or high
Serum folate ng/ml	2-10	2-10	<2	Normal or high
Serum vitamin B$_{12}$ pg/ml	200-700	200-700	Normal	<200

RBC = red blood cell; MCV = mean corpuscular volume; MCHC = mean corpuscular hemoglobin concentration and red cell indices; TIBC = total iron-binding capacity.

loss. A 30-day therapeutic trial of an oral iron supplement may be justified in women if the physical examination is normal and if the history provides a likely cause, such as frequent pregnancies or excessive menstrual blood loss. Such a course is almost never justified in men. Hypochromic microcytic anemia in a man is most commonly caused by chronic occult blood loss from the gastrointestinal tract. It usually demands careful study of stool specimens for the presence of blood and parasites as well as complete examination of the upper and lower gastrointestinal tract with roentgenograms and/or endoscopy. In the hospital, excessive blood sampling for laboratory tests may lead to iron deficiency anemia. One unit of blood contains 250 mg of iron and may require 2 to 4 months for replacement.

For treatment of iron deficiency anemia, replacement therapy with simple iron salts, such as ferrous sulfate given orally in dosages of 325 mg one to three times daily with meals, is generally quite effective. Adjunctive measures include using iron cookware, taking vitamin C with each meal (a 50-mg vitamin C tablet or a glass of orange juice), adequate intake of high-quality protein, and avoiding intake of agents known to inhibit iron absorption, such as phosphates, phytates, tannic acid in tea, and antacids.

Parenteral iron is seldom needed but is available in the form of an iron-dextran complex providing 50 mg of elemental iron per milliliter. Its use should be restricted to patients in whom serious attempts at oral therapy have failed or in whom chronic losses exceed the absorption capacity of the intestine, because fatal anaphylactic reactions have been described. Iron is a component in certain vitamin-mineral mixtures for total parenteral nutrition and is apparently safe at maintenance dosages of 1 to 2 mg/day.

Deficiency of folic acid and/or vitamin B$_{12}$

The other large category of nutritional anemia is commonly called *megaloblastic*, since deficiency of folic acid or vitamin B$_{12}$ causes accumulation of large immature red cell precursors, known as megaloblasts, in the bone marrow. A finding of arrested maturation in bone marrow smears was once the hallmark of diagnosis, but it is gradually being replaced by biochemical assessment of vitamin levels in plasma, red blood cells, and urine (see Table 2-10).

The prototype of vitamin B$_{12}$ deficiency is pernicious anemia, which strictly speaking is not a dietary deficiency because it is caused by intestinal malabsorption. Patients with pernicious anemia lack intrinsic factor (IF), a glycoprotein that is normally secreted by the parietal cells and that binds vitamin B$_{12}$. Even in the face of adequate intake of dietary sources of B$_{12}$, such as animal products, functional deficiency of vitamin B$_{12}$ can occur because of intestinal malabsorption. Either total gastrectomy or ileal resection can disrupt physiologic mechanisms of absorption. The average time of onset of megaloblastic anemia after total gastrectomy is about 4.5 years because of the large residual liver stores in most individuals.

Dietary sources of folate include most green, leafy vegetables as well as yeast, liver, beans, and peas. Dietary sources of vitamin B$_{12}$ include protein foods of animal origin. In contrast to vitamin B$_{12}$ deficiency, low dietary intake of folate is often responsible for folate deficiency anemia. Macrocytic anemia due to folate deficiency is also seen in both celiac disease and tropical sprue. In the former disorder, folate supplements are helpful, but the underlying disorder must be treated with a gluten-free diet. The latter disorder is not well understood but responds to therapy with oral folic acid, oral antibiotics, and injections of vitamin B_{12}.

The diagnosis of folic acid deficiency can be made if plasma folate level is less than 3 ng/ml; it is very likely if the value is less than 5 ng/ml. Because plasma folate fluctuates with recent dietary intake, the red cell folate is a much more reliable indicator of tissue stores. Red cell folate levels below 140 ng/ml are considered indicative of deficiency. Vitamin B_{12} deficiency is present when the plasma concentration is less than 200 pg/ml. If B_{12} is deficient, the plasma folate level may be *elevated* to 15 or 20 ng/ml. Pernicious anemia can be diagnosed by demonstrating abnormal absorption of a small oral dose of radio-active vitamin B_{12} (Schilling test) with less than 7% urinary excretion in 24 hours, provided normal uptake and excretion can be demonstrated in the presence of exogenous IF. If the latter condition is not fulfilled, intestinal malabsorption should be suspected. In cases of megaloblastic anemia, it is always desirable to establish or exclude a diagnosis of pernicious anemia, which has an absolute requirement for therapy with vitamin B_{12}. If pernicious anemia is treated with large doses of folate alone, posterolateral degeneration of the spinal cord is aggravated, although anemia may disappear.

Vitamin B_{12} repletion can be accomplished by daily parenteral injections of 100 μg of cyanocobalamin or hydroxycobalamin for several weeks. If a maintenance program is needed, as for pernicious anemia, injections of 100 μg every 2 to 4 weeks are generally adequate but should be individually adjusted according to hematologic response and blood-vitamin levels. Tablets containing 1000 μg of cyanocobalamin, used as a daily dose, are available for oral use, overcoming IF deficits by a mass action effect.

Folic acid deficiency is corrected readily in most patients with supplemental oral tablets containing 1 to 5 mg of the vitamin (pteroylglutamic acid) daily. A product containing 15 mg/mL is available for intramuscular or intravenous use. Oral dosages of up to 45 mg/day have been used for periods of several weeks without observed ill effects, but such high dosages are seldom necessary. High levels of folate supplementation may interfere with seizure control in patients receiving anticonvulsant medication.

EATING DISORDERS

Although anorexia nervosa and bulimia have been observed for decades, the prevalence of these disorders did not command the attention of the psychiatric, psychologic, and medical communities until the mid-1970s. Previously, anorexia nervosa was considered a disorder of the young, white, affluent girl or woman whose illness was a reflection of disturbed family relationships. However, within the past decade, clinicians have seen a rapid rise in the number of patients with primary eating disorders. With more cases being documented, there now remains controversy regarding etiology, diagnostic criteria, treatment, and the relationship of eating disorders to affective disorders such as depression.

Table 2-11   Diagnostic criteria for the eating disorders

ANOREXIA NERVOSA

A. Refusal to maintain body weight over a minimal normal weight for age and height, e.g., weight loss leading to maintenance of body weight 15% below that expected, or failure to make expected weight gain during period of growth, leading to body weight 15% below that expected.

B. Intense fear of gaining weight or becoming fat, even though underweight.

C. Disturbance in the way in which one's body weight, size, or shape is experienced, e.g., the person claims to "feel fat" even when emaciated, believes that one area of the body is "too fat" even when obviously underweight.

D. In girls and women, absence of at least three consecutive menstrual cycles when otherwise expected to occur (primary or secondary amenorrhea). (A woman is considered to have amenorrhea if her periods occur only following hormone administration, e.g., estrogen.)

BULIMIA NERVOSA

A. Recurrent episodes of binge eating (rapid consumption of a large amount of food in a discrete period of time).

B. A feeling of lack of control over eating behavior during the eating binges.

C. Regularly engaging in self-induced vomiting, use of laxatives or diuretics, strict dieting or fasting, or vigorous exercise in order to prevent weight gain.

D. A minimum average of two binge eating episodes a week for at least 3 months.

E. Persistent overconcern with body shape and weight.

From American Psychiatric Association. Disorders usually first evident in infancy, childhood, or adolescence. In *Diagnostic and Statistical Manual of Mental Disorders*, ed 3, Washington DC, 1987, American Psychiatric Association.

Definition and diagnosis

Anorexia nervosa is self-starvation motivated by excessive concern with weight and an irrational fear of becoming fat. Table 2-11 lists diagnostic criteria for anorexia nervosa and bulimia nervosa. People with anorexia nervosa are characterized by an extremely controlled and restrictive calorie intake and an obsessive, narrowed focus on body fat. The patient will usually deny that any problem exists and will exhibit a loss of perspective with respect to body shape.

Like anorexia nervosa, bulimia nervosa is accompanied by a preoccupation with weight and fear of becoming fat. However, unlike the anorectic person, the bulimic individual does not maintain rigid control of calorie intake. Instead, the bulimic patient binges and then purges by self-induced vomiting, use of laxatives and/or diuretics, excessive exercise, or periods of severe caloric restriction.

Formal diagnostic criteria for these disorders are outlined in Table 2-11. The following guidelines also may signal the possibility of an eating disorder:

- Amenorrhea for several consecutive months
- Complaints of fatigue, dizziness, diarrhea, headaches, or muscle cramping
- Rigid, arbitrary definitions of "fattening" foods or avoidance of certain food groups (for example, starches)
- Compulsive, intensive aerobic exercise

Etiology and associated features

Although no specific physical disorder has been implicated in the development of eating disorders, a number of demographic and psychosocial variables are consistently associated with anorectic and bulimic patients:

- Nearly all anorectic and bulimic patients are female.
- Age of onset for anorexia nervosa typically is 14 to 18 years; bulimia is most likely to develop between 18 and 22 years of age.
- Many women patients report a history of obesity.
- A family history of affective illness such as depression and/or substance abuse is common.
- Families of bulimic patients are likely to be characterized by instability and conflict. In contrast, families of anorectic patients appear closely knit but rigid.
- Because their career may depend on the ability to maintain a particular body weight, models, dancers, flight attendants, and actresses are at high risk for both anorexia nervosa and bulimia.
- The anorectic patient typically will appear rigid and controlled, whereas the bulimic patient will appear impulsive and out of control.

Medical complications

The medical complications of anorexia nervosa are similar to the metabolic and physiologic adaptations observed in starvation. These may include a slow resting heart rate and low blood pressure. The skin may be cool, and there may be loss of scalp hair and appearance of soft lanugo (fine, soft, blond) hair on the face and trunk. Hypercarotenemia and a yellowish discoloration of the skin may develop, possibly secondary to a decrease in the metabolic conversion of carotene to vitamin A, functional hypothyroidism, or consumption of large amounts of carotene-containing fruits and vegetables.

Virtually all observed endocrine changes are related to abnormalities at the level of the hypothalamus and are reversible with weight gain. The hypothalamic-pituitary-gonadal axis is the most sensitive and earliest endocrine axis to manifest changes related to anorexia. A decrease in production of follicle-stimulating hormone (FSH) and luteinizing hormone (LH), which causes decreased estrogen and progesterone levels, results in amenorrhea. Importantly, amenorrhea can occur even before significant weight loss in anorexia nervosa. Gonadotropin-releasing hormone injections can produce ovulation and menstruation, indicating that the hypothalamic-pituitary-gonadal axis is otherwise intact.

The most serious complication of anorexia nervosa relates to the cardio-vascular system and the potential for sudden death. As with any other starvation or semistarvation state, there is loss of cardiac mass which results in loss of physiologic functional capacity. For example, the predicted response of cardiac output and oxygen consumption to exercise is diminished. With this impaired functional capacity life threatening irregular heart rhythms may occur, especially when deficiencies of potassium, magnesium, and/or phosphorus are present. Thus, at this advanced stage the patient with anorexia nervosa is at significant risk for sudden death from these cardiac abnormalities.

The medical complications of bulimia, with its bingeing and purging, present a spectrum of anatomic and physiologic changes distinctly different from the adaptive changes related to starvation in the anorectic patient. Bingeing may create marked gastric dilation, and gastric rupture has been reported. A postbinge pancreatitis also may occur. Painless enlargement of the parotid glands may develop several days after a binge; in some cases it may persist and become disfiguring.

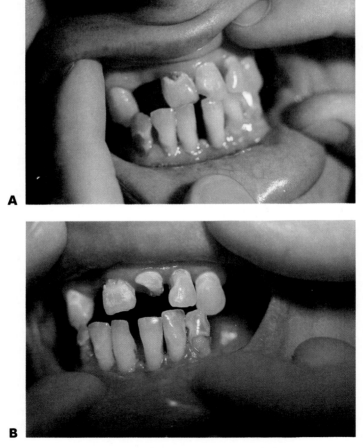

Fig. 2-7   Progression of dental erosion due to induced vomiting in a bulemic patient.

The consequences of repeated self-induced vomiting include severe erosion of the dental enamel, loss of teeth, esophagitis, hiatal hernia, esophageal tear and rupture, hypochloremic alkalosis and hypokalemia, and even shock (Figs. 2-7A and B). If ipecac is used repeatedly to induce vomiting, ipecac toxicity may develop and is associated with dysrhythmias and potentially fatal myocarditis.

Laxative abuse may result in chronic hypokalemia with renal tubular damage and cathartic dependence to maintain semblance of normal colonic activity.

Treatment

The treatment of an eating disorder depends on several factors: the severity of the problem, physical status, nature of social support, and associated psychopathology. If significant medical complications are present, the patient may require hospitalization, but in the absence of physical distress, the other factors may determine the prognosis of outpatient treatment.

Initially, symptomatic treatment may begin with weekly follow-up visits. The patient's weight should be monitored for any changes greater than a few pounds, which may indicate bingeing, semi-starvation, excessive exercise, laxative use, or diuretic use. In addition, the physician should insist that the patient maintain a food diary. Resistance to keeping such a record is a "red flag" that the patient is defensive about her eating pattern and may be experiencing binge episodes. After several visits, the physician will be in a position to evaluate the patient's attitude toward eating, preoccupation with weight loss, and resistance to change.

Whether treating the problem on an inpatient or an outpatient basis, a therapeutic alliance must be established with the patient. This is most easily accomplished by involving the patient in decision making and by setting limited goals to minimize the anxiety that will accompany weight gain.

As soon as the patient is stable, reestablishing normal eating patterns is essential. The anorectic patient will initially resist increased oral intake, but setting the expectation of improved calorie intake without requiring immediate weight gain may lessen the resistance. When self-induced vomiting is a focus of treatment, the patient may require observation for 1 to 2 hours after meals to ensure absorption of most calories and to teach him to tolerate feeling full.

Education is a critical component of the treatment process. For example, the preoccupation with food, as reported by patients, is seen by the individual as evidence that she will overeat if she eats anything. Informing the patient that thoughts about food are as much a physiological phenomenon as they are psychologic and that eating will relieve them will assist the patient in rethinking and reattributing her behavior. Similarly, food phobias can be addressed by reorienting the patient to think, "It's not what I eat, but how much," that affects weight change. The association between affective disorders and eating disorders has led to extensive research evaluating the use of antidepressant medications in the treatment of anorexia nervosa and bulimia. The results have been far more encouraging with bulimic patients than with anorectic patients. No criteria have been established for determining the usefulness of antidepressant medication in a particular case, but the presence of depressive symptoms in addition to the disrupted eating pattern may justify a trial.

The evaluation and treatment of patients with eating disorders require input from a variety of sources—psychiatry, psychology, general medicine, nutrition, and social work. The need for consistent follow-up with families and patients demands the coordination of efforts of each of these disciplines.

SELECTED READING

Obesity

Committee on Diet and Health, Food and Nutrition Board, National Research Council: *Diet and Health: Supplications for Reducing Chronic Disease Risk*. Washington, 1989, National Academy Press.

Fitzwater SL, Weinsier RL, Wooldridge NH, et al: Evaluation of long-term weight changes after a multidisciplinary weight control program. *J Am Diet Assoc* 91(4):421-426, 429, 1991.

Morgan SL. Rational weight loss programs: a clinician's guide, *J Am Coll Nutr* (3):186-194, 1989.

Wadden TA, VanItallie TB, Blackburn GL: Responsible and irresponsible use of very-low calorie diets in the treatment of obesity, *JAMA* 263(1):83-85, 1990.

Weinsier RL, Wadden TA, Ritenbaugh C, et al: Recommended therapeutic guidelines for professional weight control programs, *Am J Clin Nutr* 40(4):865-872, 1984.

Diabetes mellitus

American Diabetes Association, Inc; The American Dietetic Association: *Exchange Lists for Meal Planning*, Alexandria, and Chicago, 1986.

Kiehm TG, Anderson JW, Ward K: Beneficial effects of a high carbohydrate, high fiber diet on hyperglycemic diabetic men, *Am J Clin Nutr* 29(8):895-899, 1976.

Weinsier RL, Seeman A, Herrera MG, et al: High- and low-carbohydrate diets in diabetes mellitus: study of effects on diabetic control, insulin secretion, and blood lipids, *Ann Intern Med* 80(3):332-341, 1974.

West KM, Schneider HA, Anderson CE, Coursin DB, eds: *Diabetes mellitus in nutritional support of medical practice*, Philadelphia, 1977, Harper & Row, 278-296.

Diet, hyperlipidemia and coronary artery disease

Connor WE, Bristow JD, editors: *Coronary heart disease: prevention, complications, and treatment*, Philadelphia, 1985, Lippincott.

Lipid Research Clinics Program, The Lipid Research Clinics Coronary Primary Prevention Trial Results, *JAMA* 251(3):351-364, 1984.

NIH Consensus Development Conference Statement: Lowering blood cholesterol to prevent heart disease. *Arteriosclerosis* 5:404-412, 1985.

NIH Report of the National Cholesterol Education Program Expert Panel on Detection, Evaluation, and Treatment of High Blood Cholesterol in Adults, *Arch Intern Med* 148:36-69, 1988.

Nutrition Committee, American Heart Association: Dietary guidelines for healthy American adults: a statement for physicians and health professionals, *Circulation* 77:721A-724A, 1988.

Hypertension

National Dairy Council, An update on diet and blood pressure, *Dairy Council Digest* 57(5):25-30, 1986.

Gruchow HW, Sobocinski KA, Barboriak JJ: Alcohol, nutrient intake, and hypertension in US adults, *JAMA* 253(11):1567-1570, 1985.

Weinsier RL, Norris DJ, Birch R, et al: The relative contribution of body fat and fat pattern to blood pressure level, *Hypertension* 7(4):578-585, 1985.

Diet and cancer

Committee on Diet and Health, National Research Council (U.S.): *Diet and health: implications for reducing chronic disease risk*. Washington, 1989, National Academy Press.

Reddy BS, Cohen LA, eds: *Diet, nutrition, and cancer: a critical evaluation*, vols 1 and 2, Boca Raton, 1986, CRC Press.

Nutrition and oral health

Alvarez JO, Navia JM: Nutritional status, tooth eruption, and dental cares: a review. *Am J Clin Nutr* 49:417-426, 1989.

Navia JM: *Nutrition: pre and postnatal development*. In Alfin-Slater RB, Kritchevsky D, Myron Winick, editors: *Nutrition in dental development and disease in human nutrition—a comprehensive treatise*, vol 1, New York, Plenum, 1979, 333-362.

Nizel AE: *Nutrition in preventive dentistry: science and practice*, ed 2, Philadelphia, 1981, WB Saunders.

Pollack RL, Kravitz E: *Nutrition in Oral Health and Disease*, Philadelphia, 1985, Lea and Febiger.

Osteoporosis

Abraham GE, Grewal H: *A total dietary program emphasizing magnesium instead of calcium*: effect on the mineral density of calcaneus bone in postmenopausal women on hormonal therapy, J Rprd Med 35(5):503-507, 1990.

Barrett-Connor E: *Nutrition epidemiology: how do we know what they ate?* Am J Clin Nutr 54(1 Suppl): 182S-187S, 1991.

Committee on Diet and Health, Food and Nutrition Board, Commission on Life Sciences, National Research Council: *Diet and health*, Washington, 1989, National Academy Press.

Concensus Conference: Osteoporosis, *JAMA* 252:799, 1984.

Dubovsky J: Osteoporosis and calcium: to supplement or not to supplement, *Ala J Med Sci* 24(4):431-435, 1987.

Ettinger B, Genant HK, Cann CE: Postmenopausal bone loss is prevented by treatment with low-dosage estrogen with calcium, *Ann Intern Med* 106(1):40-45, 1987.

Food and Nutrition Board, Commission on Life Sciences, National Research Council: *Recommended dietary allowances*, ed 10 rev, Washington, 1989, National Academy Press.

Gussler JD, editor: *Osteoporosis: current concepts: report of the seventh Ross conference on medical research*, Columbus, 1987, Ross Laboratories.

Need AG, Morris HA, Cleghorn DV, et al: *Effect of salt restriction on urine hydroxyproline excretion in postmenopausal women*, Arch Intern Med 151(4):757-759, 1991.

Riggs BL, Melton LJ III: Involutional osteoporosis, *N Engl J Med* 314(26):1676-1686, 1986.

Nutritional anemias

Chanarin I: *The megaloblastic anemias*, ed 2, Oxford, England, 1979: Blackwell Scientific Publications.

Feldman EB: Nutritional anemias. In *Essentials of Clinical Nutrition*, Philadelphia, 1988, FA Davis 377-387.

Food and Nutrition Board, Commission on Life Sciences, National Research Council: *Recommended Dietary Allowances*, ed 9 rev, Washington, 1980, National Academy of Sciences/National Research Council.

Kaplan AS: Biomedical variables in the eating disorders, *Can J Psychiatry* 35(9): 745-753, 1990.

Olson RE, Broquist HP, Chichester CO, et al, editors: *Nutrition reviews present knowledge in nutrition*, ed 5, Washington, 1984, Nutrition Foundation.

Eating disorders

Bruch H: Four decades of eating disorders. In Garner DM, Garfinkel PE, editors: *Handbook of psychotherapy for anorexia nervosa and bulimia*, New York, 1985, Guilford Press, 7-18.

Casper RC: The pathophysiology of anorexia nervosa and bulimia nervosa. *Annu Rev Nutr* 6:299-316, 1986.

Garfinkel PE, Kaplan AS: Anorexia nervosa: diagnostic conceptualizations. In Brownell KD, Foreyt JP, editors: *Handbook of Eating Disorders*, New York, 1986, Basic Books, 266-282.

Hall RC, Hoffman RS, et al: Physical illness encountered in patients with eating disorders. *Psychosomatics* 30(2):174-191, 1989.

Mitchell JE, Seim HC, Colon E, et al: Medical complications and medical management of bulimia, *Ann Intern Med* 107(1):71-77, 1987.

Thurstin AH, Olson AK: Issues in the diagnosis and treatment of anorexia nervosa and bulimia. *Ala J Med Sci* 24(4):427-431, 1987.

3

Nutrition Throughout the Life Cycle

Nutritional support during pregnancy
Breast-feeding
Nutrition for infants, children, and adolescents
Nutrition and aging

NUTRITIONAL SUPPORT DURING PREGNANCY

Maternal nutritional status can influence the outcome of pregnancy, especially for women at high risk for complications. Characteristics of those at greatest risk include being nonwhite, poor, uneducated, younger than 17 or older than 35, first pregnancy, frequent pregnancies (less than 1 year apart), previous pregnancy complications, and previous fetal or infant death.

Birth weight is considered the best indicator of the newborn's health. Low birth weight is a major contributing factor in approximately two thirds of all infant deaths as well as in mental retardation. Both maternal weight and weight gain during pregnancy are positively correlated with birth weight (Table 3-1 and Fig. 3-1). Other factors influencing birth weight are maternal nutritional status, maternal age, number of pregnancies, smoking, hypertension, diabetes, and neonatal infection. The better the nutritional status of the woman entering pregnancy, the more successful the outcome.

Calorie and protein needs

During pregnancy, the mother's diet must provide the necessary nutrients for the maternal and fetal tissue being formed (Table 3-2). Calorie and protein needs are highest during the third trimester, when the fetus experiences maximal growth. The recommended daily kilocalorie allowance is 300 kcal above the nonpregnant allowance, or 40 kcal/kg of body weight, with a minimum of 36 kcal/kg. The recommended daily allowance for protein is 30 g more than for the nonpregnant woman. Recommended weight gain during pregnancy is at least 25 lb. Weight gain should be about 1 lb per month during the first trimester and 1 lb a week during the second and third trimesters. Regarding protein and energy requirements and weight gain during pregnancy, the following points are important:

- Lower weight gains are associated with lower birth weight.
- Limiting weight gain during pregnancy by dietary restriction is indicated only in cases of severe obesity.
- Weight loss is not recommended even for obese pregnant women.
- Excessive weight gain does not cause pregnancy-induced hypertension.

Table 3-1   Components of weight gain during pregnancy

Components	Weight (lb)
Infant at birth	7.5
Blood volume, maternal	4.0
Mammary tissue	3.0
Uterus and surrounding muscles	2.5
Amniotic fluid	2.0
Placenta	1.0
Maternal fat stores	5.0-10.0
Total	25.0-30.0

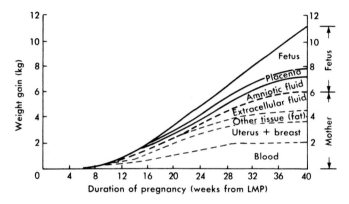

Fig. 3-1   Pattern and components of average maternal weight gain during pregnancy. LMP = last menstrual period. (From Schneider HA, Anderson CE, Coursin DB. *Nutritional support of medical practice*, Hagerstown, Md., ed 2, 1983, Harper & Row Publishers, Inc.)

Table 3-2   Nutritional guidelines during pregnancy

Food group	Daily amount
Dairy products	Equivalent to 4 cups fortified milk
Meat	6-8 oz
Grains/starches	4-5 enriched or whole-grain servings
Vegetables	Green leafy: 1-2 servings
Other	1 or more servings
Fruits	Citrus: 1-2 servings
Other	≥1 servings

Increased protein intake is needed to support the rapid growth of the fetus, placental development, enlarging maternal tissue, increased maternal blood volume, and formation of amniotic fluid. Efficient use of protein depends on adequate energy intake. Thus, if calories are reduced, protein requirements are increased.

Minerals

Edema, a result of water and sodium retention, is a normal physiological part of pregnancy that correlates with higher birth weight. If a sudden, excessive weight gain arises from edema, it could signal pregnancy-induced hypertension (PIH), but edema alone does not indicate the need for salt restriction or the use of diuretics.

Increased calcium and phosphorus are needed to promote mineralization of the fetal skeleton. The recommended calcium and phosphorus intake is approximately 400 mg higher than that for the nonpregnant woman. If dairy products are not used by the pregnant woman, calcium supplementation is recommended. With the typical American diet, the phosphorus requirement is easily met. An adequate calcium and phosphorus intake appears to lessen the incidence of PIH.

Iron is needed for the increased manufacture of hemoglobin in the mother and fetus. This is one nutrient that the fetus draws from the mother at her expense if intake in inadequate. The fetus accumulates most of its iron during the last trimester; therefore, the preterm newborn may experience iron deficiency anemia. Supplementation is generally recommended to prevent depletion of maternal iron stores and to ensure that the fetal iron stores are adequate for the first year. The recommended level of supplementation is 30 to 60 mg daily throughout pregnancy and for 2 to 3 months after delivery.

With zinc deficiency there is an increased risk of congenital malformation, an infant that is small for its gestational age, spontaneous abortion, and PIH. The recommended allowance for zinc during pregnancy is 5 mg above the level of the nonpregnant woman. This level is easily met if protein needs are met. Other minerals for which there are increased needs during pregnancy are iodine, magnesium, and copper, although supplements are usually unnecessary.

Vitamins

As with the other nutrients, vitamin needs are increased during pregnancy. With an adequate diet, the use of multivitamin supplements is not necessary, although folate supplementation is recommended. In a normal pregnancy, folate turnover is increased in the expanding maternal and fetal tissues; and folate deficiency is strongly correlated with neural tube defects in the fetus and with iron deficiency anemia.

Deficiency of vitamin B_6 in pregnant women has been reported to cause nausea and depression as well as low Apgar scores in the newborn. However, there is still controversy regarding these findings.

A deficiency of thiamin, riboflavin, or niacin may result in congenital malformation, retarded growth, and fetal death. The requirements for these nutrients are directly related to caloric intake; and since caloric intake is usually increased during pregnancy, so is the requirement for these nutrients.

The use of large doses of vitamin C for an extended period during pregnancy poses a special risk to the infant. Because it induces production of enzymes in the fetus for catabolism of the vitamin, upon delivery the newborn infant may begin to exhibit a deficient state.

Excessive intake of vitamin A may be teratogenic and cause urogenital and central nervous system malformations such as microcephaly. Vitamin D is required for calcium and phosphorus absorption and mineralization of bone tissue of the fetus, although an excess may promote neonatal hypercalcemia and abnormal skull development. Vitamin D deficiency can lead to poor tooth enamel development and hypocalcemia in the fetus. If the pregnant woman is exposed to sunlight and/or increases her dietary intake of fortified milk, the increased needs for vitamin D are generally met.

Special considerations

The pregnant adolescent is at high nutritional risk. She needs adequate energy, protein, and micronutrients to support not only her own rapid growth and maturation but also those of the rapidly growing fetus. Many of the adverse outcomes of the adolescent pregnancy are preventable through active nutrition and health care intervention. Nutritional counseling should begin as soon as possible.

Alcohol crosses the placenta to the fetus. The minimum safe level of alcohol intake for a positive pregnancy outcome has not been determined, and there is evidence that even small amounts may be harmful. Thus, the recommendation is to eliminate alcohol consumption during pregnancy. Fetal alcohol syndrome is the term used to describe the adverse effects of excessive alcohol consumption on the infant.

Characteristics of the infant with fetal alcohol syndrome include abnormalities of the eyes, nose, heart, and central nervous system; growth retardation; small head circumference; failure to thrive; and mental retardation. These characteristics are most pronounced in the babies of mothers with a long history of heavy drinking.

Pica is the persistent ingestion of unsuitable substances having little or no nutritional value. The most commonly reported practices are eating dirt, clay, or laundry starch. Although the nutritional implications of this practice are not well documented, it is speculated that ingestion of pica substances reduces the intake of essential nutrients. Other reported complications are interference with the absorption of certain minerals such as iron; lead poisoning; hemolytic anemia in the fetus; and parasitic infections. For unclear reasons, black pregnant women represent the population most likely to exhibit pica.

Pregnant women with diabetes mellitus are advised to divide their diet into several small meals throughout the day. If the diabetes is difficult to control, every meal and snack should contain protein and carbohydrate and should be given at consistent intervals each day. Intake of sucrose should be minimized.

Diabetes is defined as gestational if the carbohydrate intolerance has its onset or first recognition during pregnancy, whether or not insulin is required. Pregnant women should be screened for glucose intolerance, because undetected hyperglycemia places the fetus at greater risk for intrauterine death.

PIH is often called preeclampsia or eclampsia. Preeclampsia is characterized by hypertension, protein in the urine, and edema. Eclampsia, which is more severe, includes convulsions or coma. PIH is most likely to occur among underweight women who fail to gain appropriately during pregnancy.

Other problems, considered minor by some, that occur during pregnancy include **morning sickness,** which is usually seen in early pregnancy and is best treated with small, frequent meals, easily digested foods, and liquids between meals; **constipation,** which is best treated by increasing intake of fluids, whole grains, fruits, and vegetables rather than the use of laxatives; **hemorrhoids,** which may be aided by rest and warm baths; and **heartburn or a full feeling,** especially likely during the last trimester, which is aided by eating small, frequent meals, chewing well, and eating slowly.

BREAST-FEEDING
Recommendations and rationale

Breast-feeding is the infant feeding regimen recommended by the World Health Organization and all major national and international agencies and groups concerned with maternal and infant nutrition. The American Academy of Pediatrics recommends that infants be breast fed exclusively for the first 4 to 6 months. Their endorsement is based on the decreased morbidity in breast-fed compared with formula-fed infants, on the substantial compositional differences between human milk and commercial formula, and on the psychological and behavioral benefits to mother and child.

Human milk is the ideal nutrient source for infants; it provides immunologic protection and various growth factors expected to enhance related functional capabilities. The responsiveness of the immunologic complex in human milk to environmental stimuli and the modulation of milk composition in apparent synchrony with infant development are additional characteristics that make human milk uniquely suited to the needs of the human infant. A commercial formula that incorporates these characteristics and all human milk components with biological activity is unlikely in the near future.

Maternal status after delivery is improved by hormones released during breast-feeding. Blood loss is controlled and uterine involution is accelerated by the suckling, which induces release of oxytocin in the days after delivery. During the period of exclusive breast-feeding, ovulation is suppressed. (Breast-feeding, however, is not a reliable method of birth control as the postpartum return of ovulation may precede menses). Lactating women exhibit reduced responses to stress compared with those in nonlactating mothers. The perceived stress reduction may be modulated by the action of hormones released during breast-feeding and may be of notable benefit in the development of the mother-infant relationship.

Maternal dietary requirements

Production of human milk theoretically requires approximately 500 calories a day above the energy needed by nonpregnant women. Most lactating women, however, consume only 200 to 300 extra calories each day while producing ample quantities of milk. Many, although not all, women experience a very gradual weight loss during lactation. In addition to extra calories, breast-feeding requires approximately 20 g of additional protein and varying amounts of other nutrients.

Calcium needs are elevated during lactation; a prudent recommendation is that lactating women consume 1200 mg of calcium from dietary sources daily. Protein, calories, and calcium needs can be met through the addition of 3 to 3.5 servings of dairy products to the diet daily. For women unable to consume adequate amounts of dietary calcium, supplements (approximately 600 mg per day) are recommended to prevent bone loss. The needs for ascorbic acid, vitamin E, and folic acid are also increased during lactation and can be met with foods such as fruits, whole grains, and leafy green vegetables. Iron supplementation may be needed to replenish iron stores if the diet during pregnancy was poor in iron or if iron deficiency developed during the preceding pregnancy. Suggested eating patterns for lactating women are the same as those for pregnant women (see Table 3-2), except for the recommendation of greater milk or dairy product intake. It is important to recognize, however, that women should not be discouraged from breast-feeding because of poor eating habits. Maternal diets should be improved and nutrient supplements should be recommended when appropriate. However, milk of appropriate composition appears to be produced by women in diverse planes of nutrition.

Preparation for breast-feeding

Mothers with anatomical irregularities of the nipple (e.g., inverted or flat nipples) may have difficulty nursing their infants. Prenatal nipple examinations are advisable to identify women who should receive special attention during initiation of breast-feeding. In some cases, Hofman's exercises or nipple shells may correct flat or inverted nipples if used judiciously during the last two months of pregnancy. Nipple preparation, however, is unnecessary for most women.

Establishing lactation

Successful lactation can be achieved by maximizing early mother-infant contact; providing frequent, untimed nursings; prescribing supplemental bottles; and monitoring breast-feeding technique.

Mother-infant contact. Early and extended mother-infant contact with tactile stimulation of the nipple initiates release of lactogenic hormones, enhances bonding, and increases breast-feeding duration. Recent evidence suggests that extended physical contact between the newborn and mother also stabilizes infant respiration and heart rate and reduces blood pressure.

In European countries, in many of which breast-feeding rates exceed 90%, continuous rooming-in during hospital confinement is standard. This option is neither extensively used nor widely available (for poor mothers) in the United States, where breast-feeding rates are low.

While mother-infant contact, feeding frequency, and routine supplemental feedings can be managed through physician orders or hospital policies, physical assistance may be required to help mothers who are having difficulty placing their infants on the breast effectively. If the infant fails to take a sufficient amount of areola into the mouth, lactiferous sinuses may be emptied inefficiently, resulting in low milk intake and nipple trauma.

Latch-on is a particular problem during engorgement, which occurs on days 3 to 7 postpartum. Breast tissue may become painfully distended because of increased blood and lymph flow to the mammary glands. This condition is exacerbated by infrequent nursing or ineffective emptying of the breast. Areolar distention during engorgement can preclude the infant's effective latch-on even to women who experienced no difficulty during their hospital course.

Ideally, breast-feeding mothers should be contacted at 3 to 5 days postpartum to assess lactation status and the need for intervention. Management of engorgement includes use of moist heat and massage, expression of milk before nursings to soften the areola and to facilitate the infant's latch on, use of ice packs between nursings, and analgesics when necessary for pain.

Nursing frequencies. Frequent suckling (10 to 14 nursings per 24 hours in the first week) results in greater milk production and infant weight gain at 2 weeks postpartum. Nursing on demand is recommended, although it is important to understand that recognition of infant hunger is a learned skill. The number of nursings prompted by demand feeding depends on maternal recognition of infant hunger signals. Some instruction is helpful, particularly in view of the widespread misconception that all infants cry when they need to be fed. Unfortunately, undernourished infants are even more likely to sleep through needed feeding in an apparent effort to conserve energy. If the mother fails to detect hunger signals, or if the infant fails to give the signals, considerable weight deficit can accrue between hospital discharge and the first pediatric visit. New mothers are best advised to wake infants to feed, if necessary, to achieve an optimal high feeding frequency during the interval between hospital discharge and the first well-baby visit. Careful observation of sleeping infants will usually reveal fidgeting or hand sucking during extended sleep periods. For sleepy infants, attempted nursings during these periods will be most productive. Infant weight gain can be evaluated at the first well-baby visit, and interpretation of infant hunger signals and nursing frequency can be adjusted accordingly.

Neonatal jaundice. Breast-fed infants are more likely to experience neonatal jaundice than formula-fed infants. In the past, water supplements were prescribed prophylactically to prevent elevation in serum bilirubin concentrations. Such supplements, however, are now believed to be ineffective. Frequent breast-feeding during the immediate puerperium is associated with low serum bilirubin levels at discharge. Breast-feeding appears to stimulate the infant's gastric motility and to cause increased fecal elimination of bilirubin and reduced enterohepatic circulation of bilirubin.

When elevated serum bilirubin levels are observed in breast-fed infants, treatment may include increased nursing frequency and supplementation with formula. The added formula will increase stool volume and net bilirubin elimination, thus reducing increase in bilirubin levels associated with hypocaloric intakes. Discontinuation of breast-feeding for 1 to 3 days may aid in the differential diagnosis of human milk jaundice. If discontinuation of breast-feeding is used for diagnostic purposes, it is important that mothers be provided with the information and skills needed to maintain the development of adequate lactation during the trial period. No detrimental effects of human milk jaundice have been reported.

Reports have suggested that the use of supplemental feedings during hospitalization is associated with a shorter duration of breast-feeding than when supplemental feedings are not given. Whether supplemental feedings cause or are merely associated with added formula feedings is not clear. Prudent medical practice dictates that supplemental feedings be used only when medically indicated.

Estimating intake. Before the first well-baby visit, infant intake can be monitored for signs of inadequate intake. Danger signals for inadequate intake in the early postpartum period include infrequent bowel movements (fewer than four per day), fewer than six wet diapers per day, concentrated urine or urate crystals in the urine, fewer than seven nursings per 24 hours, persistent crying and hunger, and inability to latch-on to the breast.

During the first month of life, most breast-fed infants stool with each nursing. Thus, 10 or more small stools a day are normal in early infancy.

After the first 4 to 6 weeks, stool frequency decreases, possibly from 10 per day to 1 every 2 or 3 days in normal healthy breast-fed infants. The decrease in stool frequency is not a problem unless accompanied by behavioral symptoms such as lethargy or irritability. Stools of breast-fed infants may be yellow, brown, or green. Stool color is not diagnostic of any abnormal condition. Stools are unformed, seedy in appearance, and have an inoffensive, sweet cheese odor resulting from the high titer of *Lactobacillus bifidus* in the breast-fed infant's colon.

Maintaining lactation

Mothers who wean their infants prematurely most commonly cite an insufficient milk supply as the reason. However, both reduced milk production and cessation of lactation are usually preventable if sound physiological principles are applied.

Feeding frequency. Feeding frequency continues to be important to breast-feeding success throughout lactation. During periods termed appetite spurts, breast-fed infants may demand to be fed almost continually. Appetite spurts are reported at approximately 12 days of age, 3 to 4 weeks, and at variable intervals thereafter. The behavior resolves spontaneously within approximately 3 days if the mother increases nursings until milk production is increased. Offering formula supplements during appetite spurts undermines maternal milk production and may precipitate lactation failure.

By 4 weeks of age, exclusively breast-fed infants nurse approximately eight to nine times in 24 hours. The actual frequency may be much higher but is rarely as low as six times per 24 hours when infant growth is adequate. As lactation progresses, the mean nursing frequency drops slightly. When frequencies drop to six per 24 hours, maternal basal prolactin levels decline, and milk production may decrease. Night feedings are less common after 3 months of age, but many breast-fed infants do not sleep through the night until after weaning.

Feeding duration. The usual duration of individual feedings is 3 to 20 minutes per breast. Consistent nursing over 25 to 30 minutes per breast may indicate inadequate milk production or inappropriate latch-on. Although most infants extract 80% to 90% of the milk within 5 minutes of nursing, efficiency of milk extraction varies from infant to infant on the basis of latch-on and suckling vigor. Moreover, since milk fat is preferentially released toward the end of the feeding, arbitrary truncation of feeding times may significantly reduce caloric intake. If the mother is distressed by the long nursing durations and if infant weight gain is less than satisfactory, the mother should be referred to a lactation consultant.

Special situations

Working and breast-feeding. Infants who receive either formula or expressed human milk while their mothers are away should be introduced to bottle feeding by 3 to 4 weeks of age. Bottle-feeding skills can be maintained by giving a bottle daily or several times a week. If this is not done, the infant may refuse to nurse from a bottle by 2 to 3 months of age.

Working mothers who wish to continue exclusive breast-feeding may be advised to substitute pumping for some nursings to maintain a total of six or more breast emptyings per day. Increase in nursing frequency on weekends and holidays may be necessary to maintain milk volume. The range of appropriate nursing frequencies is broad when breast-feeding and formula feeding are combined.

Mothers may be advised to begin expressing milk 2 to 3 weeks before returning to work. Initial success is enhanced by pumping the second breast early in the morning, when milk production is at its peak, and immediately after the infant has stimulated oxytocin release by nursing the other breast. Expressed milk may be stored in glass or hard plastic containers, refrigerated immediately, and fed within a day or frozen and fed within 3 months. Some loss of immunologic components will occur if milk is frozen in polyethylene bags. Frozen milk can be thawed quickly by swirling gently under warm running water. This technique prevents the possibility that previously frozen milk will be left at room temperature for long periods during which bacteria may grow and milk fat may break down.

Occluded lactiferous ducts. Occluded lactiferous ducts, characterized by areas of localized breast tenderness, result from milk stasis secondary to infrequent or incomplete breast emptying. If left untreated, occluded ducts may precipitate mastitis. Management includes moist heat and massage and frequent nursing, beginning with the affected breast. Frequent nursing in a variety of nursing positions with concurrent breast massage is the most effective preventive technique.

Mastitis. Mastitis is an inflammation of breast connective tissue or ducts. Symptoms of mastitis include fever, body aches, and breast pain; symptoms may also include erythematous streaks or lumps in the breast. *Staphylococcus aureus* is the most common bacterial etiologic agent and *Streptococcus* is the next most common cause, although other pathogens also may cause this condition. Prompt treatment with an antistaphylococcal antibiotic is indicated for initial bouts of mastitis. Mothers should be cautioned to continue the full course (7 to 14 days) of oral antibiotic. Recurrent infection is common when mothers discontinue medication after symptoms are alleviated.

Sore nipples. Sore nipples are normal during the first week of lactation. Pain usually is most noticeable on initial latch-on and subsides after 30 seconds to a minute. Prolonged nipple pain throughout nursing and nipple pain that persists beyond the first two weeks may result from incorrect suckling, nipple trauma, or bacterial or fungal infection of the nipple. Virtually all sore nipples benefit from careful attention to rinsing, thorough drying, and 10 to 15 minutes of air exposure after nursing. Suspected bacterial infections may be treated with a topical antibiotic; the breast should be rinsed and dried before nursing. Yeast infections require simultaneous treatment of mother and infant to prevent reinfection. Mothers with persistent sore nipples may be referred to a lactation consultant.

Infant refusal to nurse. Refusal to nurse, named by some as *nursing strikes,* may occur at any time and may last several hours or even days. A variety of conditions have been associated with this sometimes abrupt behavior (for example, respiratory infections, thrush, otitis media, teething, changes in maternal diet, changes in soaps and perfumes, resumption of menses). Often such episodes are unexplained and resolve spontaneously. When no other symptoms are observed in the infant, reassurance and advice to offer quiet, soothing feeding opportunities may be the most the clinician can suggest. If normal nursing is not resumed in a reasonable time, the child should be examined to rule out underlying illness

Maternal and infant illness. Maternal or infant illness usually is compatible with breast-feeding. Exceptions include active, untreated tuberculosis and acquired immunodeficiency syndrome (AIDS) in the mother. The *Physicians' Desk Reference* is not necessarily an appropriate authority on drugs that are safe for or that preclude breast-feeding. Clinicians may contact a pharmacist who is knowledgeable about drugs and breast-feeding or use a reference that specifically addresses the topic. In considering maternal medications, it is important to take into account possible interactions with medications prescribed for the infants.

Weaning

Introduction of solid foods. Solid foods may be added to the diet when the infant is 4 to 6 months of age. The introduction of solid foods into the diet of 4- to 6-month-old exclusively breast-fed infants results in reduced milk intake despite attempts to maintain nursing frequency. During the first month, total energy intake also declines slightly. Feeding efficiency increases, and total caloric intake returns to the level achieved during exclusive breast-feeding in the second month after solids are introduced. Single-ingredient foods should be introduced first and new foods offered at intervals of no less than 5 to 7 days to enable the detection of allergies or intolerance to specific foods.

Weaning. Weaning may be initiated either by the infant or the mother and is most successful if done gradually. Nursing frequency may be decreased by one nursing every 3 to 7 days. This allows time for breast involution and decreases the possibility of engorgement and mastitis. Solid foods and/or other liquids may be offered in place of each eliminated feeding.

NUTRITION FOR INFANTS, CHILDREN, AND ADOLESCENTS

In terms of nutrition, children are not merely small adults. They not only require a balance of nutrients for body function and energy needs but also have significant requirements for growth. The intestine must absorb more per unit of body weight in children. When coupled with a child's susceptibility to certain infections, diarrhea becomes one of the most common symptoms seen in children.

Since growth velocity changes during childhood, with the most rapid rates seen during the first year and at puberty, age is a critical factor in determining nutritional needs. Figure 3-2 illustrates how energy needs change with age. Note the rapid decline in requirements during the first year and the increase at the onset of puberty, which is difficult to predict because not all children enter puberty at the same time. Thus, the figure represents only an approximation and is not intended to represent the needs of all children. The first point in Figure 3-2 represents the estimated requirements of a preterm infant if growth rate was equal to the intrauterine growth rate. This of course seldom happens, and the caloric intake of the preterm is usually less than the 130 kcal per kg per day listed. Protein estimates are illustrated in Figure 3-3, where again requirements correlate with growth rate. The accepted limit for protein intake in the infant is 4 g/kg. Less than 2 g/kg in the infant may lead to protein malnutrition.

Under normal circumstances, multivitamin and mineral supplements are not required for the growing child. However, there are some exceptions. Vitamin K supplementation for all newborn infants is routinely given as a single intramuscular dose of 0.5 to 1 mg or an oral dose of 1 to 2 mg at the time of birth to prevent hemorrhagic disease. Fluoride supplements are indicated in all children if the water supply contains less than 0.3 ppm of fluoride. The acceptable dosage is 0.25 mg per day in an infant less than two years of age, 0.5 mg per day at 2 to 3 years, and 1 mg per day up to age 16 years. Requirements for iron in the infant over 6 months of age are most likely to be met if an iron-fortified infant formula is used.

The nutrient needs of preterm infants are proportionately greater than those for term infants because of the increased demands of more rapid growth and less complete intestinal absorption. Hence, vitamin and mineral supplements are recommended for these infants.

The RDA for infants, children, and adolescents are given in Chapter 1, Tables 1-1 and 1-2.

Infant formulas. Breast-feeding is considered the best choice for feeding the normal full-term infant. (For more on breast-feeding, see pp. 54–59.) However, because not all mothers choose to breast-feed, nutritious substitutes for human milk have been developed. Formula composition has evolved over the past 50 years as our understanding of nutrient requirements, absorptive physiology, and metabolism has advanced. Today's infant formulas contain fat, carbohydrate, protein, minerals, vitamins, and water in amounts sufficient to meet the needs of a healthy, growing infant.

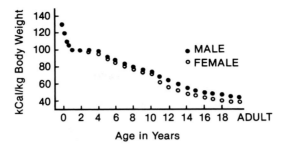

Fig. 3-2   Total energy requirements in children.

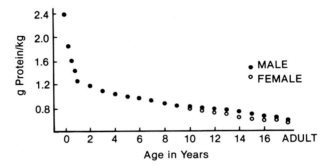

Fig. 3-3   Safe levels of protein intake in children.

Lactose, the disaccharide found in almost all mammalian milk, is the most common sugar found in infant formula. It is absorbed less efficiently than other sugars, allowing a small amount to enter the distal bowel, where it is fermented by intestinal bacteria, resulting in a slightly lower pH in the intestinal lumen. This change appears to favor the growth of acidophilic bacteria at the expense of less favorable or pathogenic bacteria. Lactose also seems to enhance the absorption of calcium. Although lactose intolerance in infants can result from gastroenteritis, primary or genetic, intolerance usually does not appear until age 4 or 5 years and starts very gradually.

Sucrose- or starch-based formulas are indicated for the infant with lactose intolerance. These sugars are more efficiently absorbed than lactose, so they do not have the beneficial effects described above.

Most infant formulas use vegetable oil as their source of fat. These oils are generally polyunsaturated and cholesterol free. This is distinctly different from human milk, which contains saturated fat and cholesterol. Whether this has any physiologic significance is unknown. Some special formulas contain medium-chain triglycerides.

Casein traditionally has been the protein used in largest quantities in infant formula, because most have a cow-milk base. Casein is precipitable in acid and makes up 80% of the protein in cow milk. Human milk contains only 20% of its protein as casein and the rest as whey protein. Whey protein is soluble in acid and is composed primarily of lactalbumin and lactoglobulin. Recently whey protein has been used extensively in infant formulas because it does not form curd in the acid environment of the stomach and is emptied quickly from the stomach.

Both casein and whey protein are known to cause allergic reactions in some infants. Formulas based on soy isolate as the protein source were developed for these infants. It is now known, however, that at least 20% of infants allergic to casein also are allergic to soy. Hydrolyzed casein is the protein of choice in casein hypersensitivity. Casein is enzymatically hydrolyzed to make a mixture of amino acids and peptides of various chain lengths, which are not allergenic.

Solid foods. Solid foods should be introduced when the infant is approximately 4 to 6 months old. Before this time, the feeding of solids is made difficult by the presence of the extrusor reflex, a forward thrusting of the tongue that forces the object placed on it out of the mouth. The hazards of premature introduction of solid foods include fluid and electrolyte abnormalities from an excess renal solute load and overfeeding with subsequent obesity.

Because iron stores are limited in the newborn infant, the first solid food recommended is iron-fortified infant cereal. Beyond this, the sequence of introduction of solid foods tends to be dictated more by tradition than by physiology. The following schedule is traditional:

Month	Food Items
1-4	Breast milk or formula only
4-6	Iron-fortified cereal
6-7	Strained fruits; begin introducing cup
7-8	Strained vegetables
8-9	Start finger foods and chopped (junior) foods
9	Meats, citrus juice
10	Bite-sized cooked foods
12	All table foods

Intestinal solute load. Because the intestine is a semipermeable membrane, rapid introduction of a high-solute (osmolar) load results in a shift of water from the bloodstream into the lumen of the bowel, causing diarrhea. Because the infant is particularly prone to osmotic diarrhea, care must be taken not to select a formula with high osmolality. If an elemental formula with a high osmolality must be used, it should be carefully introduced to allow the bowel to adapt. The solute load of various formulas with reference to human milk is listed in Table 3-3.

Renal solute load. Certain elements of our diet require excretion by the kidneys, either because they are metabolic waste products or because they are ingested in quantities greater than are required by the body. Water is required to excrete these materials, which include urea, sodium, potassium, chloride, and to a lesser extent sulfates and phosphates. For each gram of protein ingested, approximately 4 mOsm of solute are produced in the form of urea. Because our bodies tend to stay in balance with regard to sodium, potassium, and chloride,

Table 3-3   Osmolarity of human milk and infant formulas

Human milk	275 mOsm/L
Similac	290 mOsm/L
Enfamil	300 mOsm/L
SMA	300 mOsm/L
Pregestimil	310 mOsm/L
Nutramigen	290 mOsm/L
Lofenalac	320 mOsm/L

for each milliequivalent of these substances ingested, a milliosmol of solute must be excreted.

Because of immaturity, the infant kidney can only concentrate urine to an osmolality of about 600 mOsm/L. If an infant is fed 1 L of cow milk, which contains a potential renal solute load of 275 mOsm/L, almost half of the water ingested in the milk will be required to excrete the solute. The actual volume of water required is calculated as follows:

$$275 \text{ mOsm}/600 \text{ mOsm} \times 1000 \text{ ml} = 458 \text{ ml}$$

Because insensible water loss (i.e., usual loss through the lungs, skin, and urine) requires at least half of the ingested water of an infant, nothing is left to cover increased loss of water in situations such as sweating, diarrhea, fever, and so on. This makes the infant very vulnerable to fluid and electrolyte abnormalities if fed substances with a high renal solute load such as cow milk.

The premature infant. Special formulas are available for feeding the premature infant with very low birth weight. They are recommended until the infant achieves a body weight of approximately 1.8 kg. The composition of these formulas differs markedly from that of human milk. In general, they have a higher protein content, contain significant amounts of medium-chain triglycerides, are low in lactose, and contain slightly more sodium.

When the infant with very low birth weight is fed human milk, requirements for normal growth may not be met. On the other hand, human milk may provide immunological protection for the premature infant. For this reason, methods are available to fortify human milk for the feeding of the premature infant. In the meantime, the following guidelines are recommended:

- Nasogastric tube feeding is begun, first with sterile water.
- Human milk can then be fed by continuous nasogastric drip (syringe pumps are recommended), especially if the infant weighs less than 1300 g.
- When full feeding volume is achieved, fortification of the human milk is instituted. After the infant reaches a weight of 1600 to 1800 g, breast- or bottle-feeding is introduced, and when fed entirely by nipple, fortification is discontinued.
- Until the infant's condition is stable, close monitoring of nutritional status is critical, including blood levels of electrolytes, hemoglobin, urea nitrogen, and albumin.

Feeding the child. During the second year of life, children begin taking some initiative in food selection. The use of finger foods, spoons, and cups should be encouraged to help continue the development of manual dexterity and coordination.

Three meals and two snacks should be offered each day, and parents should realize that food intake will vary from day to day. Increasing the variety of tastes, colors, textures, and temperatures of foods from the basic four food groups will help maintain adequate intake. Foods likely to be aspirated should be avoided, including hot dogs, nuts, grapes, round candies, popcorn, and raw carrots.

Ages 2 through 5 years are characterized by an increasingly active participation in family life. Meals become important socially as well as nutritionally. A regular meal schedule should be developed to meet the increasing energy needs of the child.

When the child starts school, many changes occur. The school schedule reinforces limit setting; and since lunch is eaten at school, added choices need to be made. Children need to eat foods different from those at home, and school lunch offers this opportunity. An after-school snack may be needed but should not replace or interfere with the evening meal.

As the child gets older, pressures and temptations to replace the school lunch with other purchases may be great. Competitive sports also may influence the child's eating habits. Nutrition programs designed for older children or for professional athletes should not be applied to young children.

Feeding the adolescent. The adolescent's food habits differ from those of any other age group and are characterized by an increasing tendency toward skipping meals, snacking, dieting, vegetarianism, and inappropriate consumption of fast foods. These behaviors often can be explained by the teen's newly found independence, difficulty in accepting existing values, poor body image, search for self-identity, peer acceptance, and conformity of life-style. An understanding of these factors is necessary for proper counseling of a teenager about diet.

Particular care needs to be taken to provide adequate intake of calcium, iron, and zinc, which frequently are marginal in the adolescent diet. The vegetarian teenager who does not eat eggs, cheese, or other dairy products is at increased risk for deficiencies of vitamins D and B_{12}, calcium, iron, zinc, and perhaps other trace metals. Obesity, anorexia nervosa, and bulimia are commonly found in the adolescent and are best handled with professional advice. (For more on eating disorders, see Chapter 2.)

NUTRITION AND AGING

As people age, their energy requirements are less, and they tend to eat less. Unless food is carefully selected, the intake of essential micronutrients may fall below desired levels. This is compounded by social and economic conditions of poverty, loneliness, and chronic diseases that can lead to further dietary inadequacies. Consequently, the elderly constitute a nutritionally vulnerable population.

With aging there is a decrease in body weight and a change in body composition, reflected by a decrease in lean body mass and a relative increase in fat. It is estimated that there is a 6% decrement in lean body mass, mainly skeletal muscle, with each decade after age 30. The 1983 Metropolitan Life Insurance Reference Weights have been applied to populations older than 60 years of age. Weights of 20% above or below these reference standards may identify people who are at risk for obesity or malnutrition.

Although energy requirements decline with age, largely because of a sedentary existence, basal calorie expenditure per day falls only slightly due to aging. The declining need for calories is recognized by the Recommended Daily Allowance (RDA), which suggests that men between 25 and 50 years of age consume 2900 kcal per day, whereas the recommendation for men older than 50 is 2300 kcal (see Table 1-1). For women aged 25 to 50, an intake of 2200 kcal is recommended, but for women 50 and older, only 1900 kcal is indicated.

Dietary surveys and biochemical assessments of Americans 65 years of age and older have indicated a number of dietary inadequacies, including thiamin, riboflavin, vitamin C, vitamin B_6, vitamin C, folate, calcium, and zinc. Mental function tests conducted on healthy people older than 60 years have shown a relationship of poor performance to low nutritional status in riboflavin, folate, vitamin C, and vitamin B_{12}.

Nutrient recommendations

In general, the recommended amounts of vitamins for the elderly are the same as for adults younger than 50 years. Slight reductions are indicated for thiamin, riboflavin, and niacin, reflecting reduced energy expenditure. Although the data are limited, thiamin and riboflavin requirements do not appear to increase with age. The recommended intake of iron is reduced to 10 mg per day for women because of cessation of menstruation. Protein requirements do not appear to decrease with age.

These dietary recommendations are based on limited information; little is known about the actual declines or increases in nutrient needs that correspond with the aging process. For example, the RDA for calcium is 800 mg per day for women. Calcium balance studies of postmenopausal women indicate that their calcium requirements are considerably higher, possibly by at least 50%.

Iron. A dietary deficiency in iron does not appear to be a general consequence of aging, because the incidence of iron deficiency in the elderly is usually low. When it does occur, it is commonly associated with a loss of blood from the gastrointestinal tract. The hemoglobin and hematocrit standards used in younger people do not appear to be suitable for application to older populations. Consequently, the use of these standards may suggest an apparent presence of anemia in the elderly.

Zinc. Information regarding the dietary intake of zinc suggests that it may be low in the elderly. This is reflected in the impaired taste acuity and low blood zinc levels found in the elderly.

Calcium. Osteomalacia, a bone condition associated with a deficiency of vitamin D and calcium, may occur in the elderly, in whom calcium is frequently less efficiently absorbed and in whom increased calcium is needed to achieve calcium balance. The elderly tend to have a lower exposure to sunlight, which results in a reduced synthesis of vitamin D in their skin. Calcium levels in the elderly often fall because of the lower intake of milk, dairy products, and other calcium sources. (Also see Osteoporosis, Chapter 2.)

Vitamin A. Vitamin A deficiency has seldom been observed in the elderly, although low dietary intake of vitamin A has been reported for this age group. However, few studies have investigated the occurrence of night blindness and impaired adaptation to the dark in the elderly.

Vitamin C. Elderly people with dental problems frequently avoid eating fruits and vegetables that could serve as a source of vitamin C. Hence, low blood vitamin C levels and scurvy are observed in the elderly. These conditions usually respond to vitamin supplements.

Thiamin. Dietary studies suggest that thiamin intake is often below desirable levels in a significant segment of the elderly population, but clinical cases of thiamin deficiency in the form of beriberi are rare in the United States. However, cases are encountered among elderly alcoholics.

Folate. Folate intake and nutritional status have been considered adequate for most elderly people. Nevertheless, folate deficiency may be observed in certain segments of the elderly population, such as those hospitalized or institutionalized, those with low incomes, those receiving certain medications that antagonize folate metabolism, those with impaired absorption, and those with alcoholism. Alcohol has a marked effect on folate metabolism, because it interrupts the enterohepatic circulation of folate, interfaces with its absorption, and causes an increase in the urinary excretion of this vitamin. Folate deficiency may be observed frequently in low-income, urban, elderly people in association with poor dietary habits and low intake of folate.

Vitamin B$_{12}$. Most cases of vitamin B$_{12}$ deficiency observed in the United States are the result of impaired absorption of the vitamin due to pernicious anemia. (See Nutritional Anemias, Chapter 2.) Latent pernicious anemia has been observed in the elderly, but a decline in the absorption of vitamin B$_{12}$ with age has not been established.

Influencing factors

Malnutrition may occur among the elderly as a result of various factors: fixed income; altered food selection and intake due to loss of teeth and reduced sense of taste and smell; use of medications; psychological depression and loneliness resulting from loss of spouse and friends; immobility; effects of declining health or chronic diseases; inability to prepare their own food; and alcoholism.

People older than 65 years represent the population group with the highest risk of illness and disability. It has been estimated that 85% of this group have some form of chronic disease that may be related to inadequate nutrition or overnutrition. Both hypokalemia and hyperkalemia occur more frequently in older people than in the young. Diuretic therapy is the most frequent cause of hypokalemia; hyperkalemia is usually observed only in patients with impaired renal function. Biochemical measurements often indicate that subclinical deficiencies of water-soluble vitamins are common among the elderly. The significance of these observations is not certain, but the deficiencies may be the cause of such symptoms as loss of appetite, malaise, insomnia, and increased irritability frequently reported in the elderly. Superimposed conditions such as surgery, infection, and trauma may precipitate clinical deficiencies.

SELECTED READING

Nutritional support during pregnancy

Board of Directors, American Diabetes Association: Position statement on diabetes in pregnancy, *Diabetes* 34:123-126, 1985.

Committee on Maternal Nutrition, National Academy of Sciences: *Maternal nutrition and the course of pregnancy,* Washington, 1970, National Academy of Sciences.

Whitney EN, Cataldo CB, Rolfes SR: *Mother and infant.* In Cataldo CB, editor: *Understanding normal and clinical nutrition,* St. Paul, 1987, West Publishing, 491-511.

Worthington-Roberts BS: *Nutrition in pregnancy and lactation,* ed 3, St. Louis, 1985, Times Mirror/ Mosby College Publishing.

Breast-feeding

Anderson GC: Risk in mother-infant separation postbirth, *Image: J Nurse Scholarship* 21(4):196-199, 1989.

Cunningham AS, Jelliffe DB, Jelliffe EF: Breast-feeding and health in the 1980s: a global epidemiologic review, *J Pediatr* 118(5):659-666, 1991.

DeCarvalho M, Hall M, Harvey D: Effects of water supplementation on physiological jaundice in breast-fed babies, *Arch Dis Child* 56:568-569, 1981.

Freed GL, Landers S, Schanler RJ. Practical Guide to Successful Breastfeeding Management, *American Journal of Diseases of Children* 145(8):917-921, 1991.

Garza C, Hopkinson JM: *Physiology of lactation.* In Tsang R, Nichols BL, editor: *Nutrition during infancy,* Philadelphia, 1988, C.V. Mosby, 20-34.

Garza C, Hopkinson J, Schanler RJ: *Human milk banking.* In Morris FH, editor: *Human milk in infant nutrition and health,* Springfield, 1986, Charles C Thomas, 225-255.

Hopkinson JM, Garza C: *Management of breastfeeding.* In Tsang R, Nichols BL, editors: *Nutrition during infancy,* Philadelphia, 1988, C.V. Mosby, 298-313.

Lawrence RA: *Breastfeeding: a guide for the medical profession,* ed 3, St. Louis, 1989, CV Mosby.

Neifert MR, Seacat JM: *A guide to successful breastfeeding, Contemp Pediatr* 3:26-45, 1986.

Nutrition for infants, children, and adolescents

Committee on Nutrition: *Pediatric nutrition handbook,* ed 2, Elk Grove Village, 1985, Academy of Pediatrics.

Fomon SJ, Filer LJ Jr, Anderson TA, et al: Recommendations for feeding normal infants, *Pediatrics* 63(1):52-59, 1979.

Grand RJ, Stuphen JL, Dietz WH: *Pediatric nutrition, theory and practice,* Stoneham, 1987, Butterworth.

Klish WJ: Special infant formulas, *Pediatrics in review* 12(2):55-62, 1990.

Nutrition and aging

Armbrecht HJ, Prendergast JM, Coe RM, editors: *Nutritional intervention in the aging process,* New York, 1984, Springer-Verlag.

Chen LH, editor: *Nutritional aspects of aging,* vol 1, Boca Raton, Fla, 1986, CRC Press.

Feldman EB, editor: *Nutrition in the middle and later years,* Boston, 1983, Wright-PSG.

Hutchinson ML, Munro HN, editors: *Nutrition and aging,* Orlando, 1986, Academic Press.

Roe DA: *Geriatric nutrition,* Englewood Cliffs, NJ, 1983, Prentice-Hall.

4

Case Studies

CASE
STUDY **1** *Obesity*

A 26-year-old woman with mild diabetes and obesity has been on a carbohydrate-restricted, high-fat, high-protein diet to lose weight. At her most recent clinic visit, her weight and height were 91 kg and 152 cm, respectively (200 lb and 5 feet). Laboratory results showed a blood cholesterol level of 230 mg/dl and a urine test positive for ketones but negative for sugar.

TRUE or FALSE   it is reasonable to assume that:
1. Her elevated blood cholesterol level is a direct result of her obesity.
2. Her blood uric acid level is elevated.
3. Her diabetes may well be associated with her excessive body weight.
4. The ketones in the urine suggest that she was in fact fasting for at least 3 days before the laboratory examination.
5. This diet approach is appropriate for an obese patient with diabetes because of its low carbohydrate content.

CASE
STUDY **2** *Hyperlipidemia and Diabetes*

A 44-year-old man with juvenile-onset insulin-dependent diabetes mellitus, which was generally poorly controlled, was seen for worsening symptoms of intermittent cramping in the legs due to inadequate blood flow.

Physical examination. He was of normal weight but evidently in overall poor physical condition. Over his elbows, extensor surfaces of the forearms, and knees were raised, yellowish, firm papules (Fig. 4-1). Blood flow to the feet was poor.

Laboratory data. Fasting blood glucose was 305 mg/dl (with a comment from the laboratory that the whole blood looked like cream of tomato soup). In the same blood sample, serum cholesterol was 860 and triglycerides 10,000 mg/dl. A separate sample of serum, allowed to stand overnight, revealed turbidity with a creamy layer on top.

TRUE or FALSE   appropriate considerations at this time include the following:

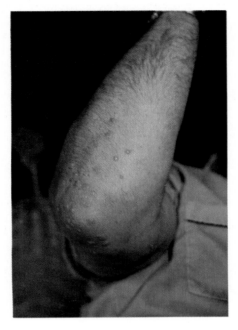

Fig. 4-1 Eruptive xanthomas in a diabetic patient with hyperlipidemia.

1. Close examination of the eyegrounds will most likely reveal lipemia (creamy appearance) of the retinal vessels.
2. On the basis of his circulating lipid levels alone, it can be surmised that his low-density lipoprotein cholesterol level will be elevated.
3. Juvenile onset of his diabetes goes along with this being a type I pattern of hyperlipoproteinemia.
4. The skin eruptions indicate that this is a true genetic form of hyperlipoproteinemia.

Reasonable considerations regarding his treatment at this time include which of the following?

5. Because of the severity of his condition, he will probably require drug therapy for the lipid abnormality.
6. Starches taken in the unrefined form to increase fiber intake may facilitate a reduced insulin requirement.
7. Alcohol intake, which may increase high-density lipoprotein cholesterol, need not be especially restricted if enjoyed by this patient.

See appendix for answers and discussion.

PART TWO

NUTRIENTS AND THE METABOLIC PROCESS

This section presents the macronutrients and micronutrients, including vitamins, minerals, water, protein, carbohydrate, fat, and energy. Sections outlining their physiology and biochemical pathways, absorption, metabolism and excretion, United States Recommended Dietary Allowance (RDA), food sources, signs of deficiency, and effects of large doses are included for easy reference. (See Tables 1-1 and 1-2).

Nutrient deficiencies and excesses

Nutrient deficiencies occur by mechanisms of
- Low nutrient intake
- Inadequate absorption
- Inadequate utilization
- Increased requirements
- Increased excretion
- Increased distribution

Although nutrient deficiencies are commonly thought to be prevalent only in underdeveloped countries, certain groups in developed countries also are at high risk.

Conditions of nutrient excess may occur unknowingly through food ingestion (e.g., vitamin A toxicity from excess liver consumption) or knowingly through the ingestion of supplements.

Megadose vitamin therapy is mandated in certain vitamin-dependent genetic diseases, in diseases associated with defective vitamin transport across cell membranes, and as an antidote to antivitamin drugs. Megadose vitamin therapy for the treatment of other medical problems (e.g., the common cold) merits further scientific scrutiny and research, because megadoses of certain vitamins are associated with a low benefit-to-risk ratio and with toxicity.

5

Macronutrients

Energy
Proteins and amino acids
Fats
Carbohydrates and fiber
Water and electrolytes

ENERGY

Energy is needed for metabolic processes that support physical activity, growth, pregnancy, and lactation. Energy allowances are expressed in terms of the physiologically available or metabolizable energy provision of foods actually eaten. Energy allowances, or energy content of foods, are expressed in terms of kilocalories or the international unit of energy, the joule; 1 kcal is equal to 4.184 kJ. The Atwater energy conversion factors for food components are used to establish the energy content of diets. For carbohydrates and protein, a value of 4 kcal/g is used for each. For fats, a value of 9 kcal/g is used, while for ethanol (alcohol) a value of 7 kcal/g (5.6 kcal/ml) is used.

Basal energy expenditure (BEE) required for metabolic processes at rest can be estimated from the following Harris-Benedict equations (where W = weight in kg, H = height in cm, and A = age in years).

For men:

$$BEE(kcal/day) = 66.47 + 13.75(W) + 5.00(H) - 6.76(A)$$

For women:

$$BEE(kcal/day) = 655.10 + 9.46(W) + 1.86(H) - 4.68(A)$$

Basal energy expenditure is estimated to increase by 20% for routine activity and by an additional 10% to 30% for patients with multiple fractures, 20% to 50% for patients with sepsis, and 90% to 100% for patients with burn injury. See Chapter 11 for further discussion.

Energy allowances are made in general terms at a level considered to be in agreement with good health of the average person. This requires consideration of differences in energy needs associated with age, activity, sex, body size, climate, pregnancy, and lactation. Precise measurement of energy balance is not always feasible. Consequently, energy requirements in RDAs are expressed as average needs for categories of individuals, recognizing that maintenance of desirable body weight throughout adult life is dependent upon energy balance. Recommended levels of intake are given in the RDA, Table 1-1.

PROTEINS AND AMINO ACIDS

The body is in a dynamic state, with proteins and other nitrogenous compounds being degraded and resynthesized continuously. With no special storage form of protein, the body requires a continuous intake of protein to replace the amino acids lost. Dietary protein serves as the source of the 20 amino acids commonly found in tissues. Nine of these amino acids (tryptophan, histidine, lysine, leucine, isoleucine, valine, threonine, phenylalanine, and methionine) are essential for humans and cannot be synthesized in the body. Histidine is required during periods of growth. Cystine can be synthesized from methionine, and tyrosine can be synthesized from phenylalanine. The remaining amino acids can be readily formed by the body and are considered nonessential amino acids.

Except for the branched-chain amino acids, the liver is the main site for the metabolism of amino acids. The branched-chain amino acids (valine, leucine, and isoleucine) are degraded mainly in peripheral tissues, particularly the skeletal muscle, but also by the kidneys and adipose tissue. In muscle and adipose tissue, the metabolism of the branched-chain amino acids is coupled to the release of glutamine and alanine. These amino acids function as carriers of ammonia groups (NH_2) to the liver, where the nitrogen may be converted into urea. In starvation or fasting, the release of alanine and glutamine provide for gluconeogenesis to assist in the maintenance of blood-sugar concentrations. In addition to alanine, other glycogenic amino acids are glycine, valine, cystine, serine, aspartic acid, asparagine, threonine, methionine, glutamine, glutamic acid, proline, arginine, and histidine. Tryptophan, tyrosine, phenylalanine, and isoleucine are partially glycogenic. Leucine and lysine are ketogenic amino acids, because they directly produce acetyl CoA or acetoacetate. Tyrosine, phenylalanine, and isoleucine are partially ketogenic, because only a portion of their carbon atoms contribute to ketogenesis.

The aromatic amino acids serve also as precursors of hormones. Tryptophan is converted to serotonin, and tyrosine is a precursor of thyroxine and the catecholamines epinephrine and norepinephrine.

The dietary allowance for proteins is 0.8 g/kg of body weight per day. Additional adjustments, as shown in Table 1-1, are made for children and pregnant and lactating women.

FATS

About 40% of the calories in the U.S. diet are derived from fat, which has a caloric value of 9 kcal/g. Dietary fat in foods occurs as a heterogeneous mixture of lipids, which consist mostly of triglycerides. Food fats also contain small amounts of phospholipids, cholesterol, sphingolipids, glycolipids, and phytosterols. Fat in the average diet is composed of approximately 35% saturated fatty acids, 40% monosaturated fatty acids, and 15% polyunsaturated fatty acids. In addition to providing a substantial proportion of energy in the diet, fats furnish essential fatty acids, serve as a carrier for fat-soluble vitamins and for food flavors, and give food desirable texture. Most fats, of either vegetable or animal origin, are readily digested and absorbed by the normal person. Less than 5% are unabsorbed and excreted in the feces.

The essential fatty acids are linoleic acid, linolenic acid, and arachidonic acid. These fatty acids or their metabolites serve as precursors for prostaglandins, thromboxanes, prostacyclins, and leukotrienes.

The requirement for essential fatty acids has not been fully defined. For populations consuming relatively low-fat diets (fat <25% of calories), a minimum of 3% of energy should be provided from linoleic acid. For those consuming diets high in fat, a higher intake may have beneficial effects. Health organizations have recommended that the total fat intake in the U.S. diet not exceed 30% of total calories. Of this, approximately one fourth to one third should be polyunsaturated fatty acids. Vegetable oils are usually a rich source of polyunsaturated fatty acids.

A dietary deficiency of essential fatty acids is rare in the adult human, but it has been observed with the use of prolonged fat-free parenteral nutrition. A deficiency can be diagnosed by analysis of the fatty acids present in plasma or red cell membranes.

The transport of lipids in circulation is discussed in Chapter 2, Section 3.

CARBOHYDRATES AND FIBER

Although carbohydrates are not essential in the same sense as the essential amino acids and fatty acids, they are our most important source of dietary energy. Each gram of carbohydrate provides approximately 4 kcal. A variety of fuels can serve as energy for most tissues, but the brain, red blood cells, and the renal medulla are normally dependent upon carbohydrates, although with extended starvation, the brain resorts to use of ketone bodies that are formed from fatty acids. Carbohydrates able to be metabolized can be easily converted into glucose, but gluconeogenesis from fats or proteins is limited to the glycerol parts of fats and the glycogenic amino acids. Carbohydrates exist in the diet in two types: (1) available carbohydrates that are digested, absorbed, and used in the body (monosaccharides such as glucose and fructose; disaccharides such as sucrose, lactose, and maltose; polysaccharides such as starches, dextrins, and glycogen) and (2) unavailable carbohydrates (such as dietary fiber).

Lactose is present exclusively in milk, and its utilization depends on lactase action in the intestine for hydrolysis to glucose and galactose. In some populations, such as orientals and blacks, many adults have a lactase deficiency and are lactose-intolerant. Although there is no specific dietary requirement for carbohydrate, it is suggested that about 50% to 60% of the caloric intake should be derived from available carbohydrates. Restriction of carbohydrate in the diet to less than 60 g/day is likely to lead to ketosis, excessive breakdown of tissue proteins, loss of cations (especially sodium), and dehydration.

The unavailable carbohydrates, primarily fiber, provide bulk in the diet and aid in elimination. Fibers represent a diverse variety of polysaccharides, mainly structural components of plant cells, which include cellulose, hemicellulose, pectins, and lignins. Although dietary fiber has no demonstrated metabolic requirement, it appears that the incidence of certain diseases, such as cardiovascular disease, diverticulosis, colon cancer, and diabetes, is inversely related to dietary fiber consumption.

Different types of plant fibers have different effects. Wheat bran, for example, has an effect on stool weight, but no effect on serum cholesterol. Pectin and oat bran have little effect on stool weight, but serum cholesterol may be lowered. The fiber intake in U.S. diets averages about 10 to 20 g/day, although it is recommended that the intake be closer to 20 to 35 g/day.

WATER AND ELECTROLYTES

Salt and water

Total body water constitutes about 60% of body weight, two thirds of which is distributed in intracellular fluid and one third in extracellular fluid. Of the extracellular fluid, three fourths is found in the interstitial fluid and one fourth in plasma. Abnormalities of extracellular fluid volume are generally caused by net gains or losses of sodium and an accompanying gain or loss of water. Volume depletion may result from unreplaced losses such as with prolonged sweating, vomiting, diarrhea, or burn injury. Fluid volume excess tends to result from diseases that prevent normal excretion of sodium and water such as kidney or heart failure. However, no laboratory tests accurately predict the degree of the volume deficit or excess; and serum sodium concentration is not a guide to volume status because it reflects only the relationship between total body water and sodium. That is, changes in sodium concentration tend to be corrected even at the expense of temporary distortion in volume.

Although a multitude of factors determine water requirements, under ordinary circumstances a reasonable allowance is 1 ml/kcal for adults and 1.5 ml/kcal for infants. (Sodium requirements are described in Chapter 2, p. 30.)

Potassium

Sodium and potassium have inverse relationships in terms of their distribution. Potassium is the primary intracellular cation with only 2% found in the extracellular fluid. Over 90% of ingested potassium is absorbed. The kidney is primarily responsible for maintaining potassium balance, and wide variations in intake are not reflected in changes in plasma concentration if there is normal renal function. Low serum levels usually reflect total body potassium deficits of over 200 mEq.

Potassium is widely distributed in foods. Good sources include meat, milk, and fruits. Usual adult intake ranges from 2 to 6 g/day (50 to 150 mEq). The higher level of intake appears beneficial in terms of blood pressure control (see "Hypertension" in Chapter 2). In healthy individuals, toxicity can result from rapid intakes of over 12 g/m² of surface area per day (about 18 g for an adult). (Potassium requirements are described in Chapter 2, p. 30).

6

Vitamins

Vitamin A
Vitamin B$_6$
Vitamin B$_{12}$
Vitamin C (Ascorbic Acid)
Vitamin D
Vitamin E
Vitamin K
Biotin
Folic Acid, Folate
Vitamin B$_3$ (Niacin)
Pantothenic Acid
Vitamin B$_2$ (Riboflavin)
Vitamin B$_1$ (Thiamin)

Vitamin A

Physiology and biochemical pathways

Vitamin A deficiency, expressed commonly as night blindness and keratomalacia (softening of the cornea), remains a major problem in many areas of the world, particularly in Southeast Asia. Young children are most likely to be affected. Both the retinol and carotenoids in the diet must be considered when determining the adequacy of vitamin A intake. In individuals consuming primarily plant foods, β-carotene and other vitamin A precursors, upon conversion to retinol, represent the major source of vitamin A in the diet. Vitamin A functions in vision in the form of retinol, is necessary for growth and differentiation of epithelial tissue, and is required for reproduction, embryonic development, and bone growth.

Absorption

Most of the β-carotene and other provitamin A precursors in the diet are normally cleaved within the mucosal cells of the duodenum and jejunum. The retinaldehyde formed from the cleavage is reduced to form retinol, is esterified, and is then transported via the lymph to the liver. Retinol is either stored in the liver or transported by plasma retinol–binding protein to active tissue sites. Protein-calorie malnutrition and zinc deficiency may impair the absorption, transport, and metabolism of vitamin A. The absorption of retinol and β-carotene is reduced in diseases that cause fat malabsorption, such as celiac disease. Retinol storage and transport are impaired in liver disease.

Metabolism and excretion

Vitamin A in the body is destroyed at a fairly steady rate, and the metabolites are excreted in the urine. Oxidized products of the vitamin are largely excreted in the bile, partly as β-glucuronides. Part of the biliary retinol β-glucuronide is reabsorbed and transported back to the liver. Retinaldehyde and retinol are reversibly interconverted. Retinaldehyde is converted to retinoic acid, which has biological activity in growth and in cell differentiation but not in reproduction or vision. The majority of the vitamin A in the body is stored in the liver.

Recommended dietary allowance and nutrient interactions

Because of the ability of β-carotene and certain other carotenoids to serve as precursors of vitamin A, requirements are expressed in terms of retinol equivalents (RE), where 1 RE equals 1 μg of retinol. For this purpose, 6 μg of β-carotene and 12 μg of other provitamin A carotenoids are equivalent to 1 μg of retinol. 1 RE equals 3.33 IU (international units) of vitamin A activity from retinol and 10 IU vitamin A activity from β-carotene. Because carotenoid and preformed vitamin A make up approximately 25% and 75% of the diet, respectively, an average value is 1 RE equals 5 IU. The recommended allowance for vitamin A as retinol equivalents is given in Table 1-1.

Food sources

Vitamin A is found in liver, butter, cheese, egg yolk, margarine, dried milk, cream, kidneys, and fortified milk, with less present in fish and seafoods. Carrots, spinach and other greens, mangoes, apricots, peaches, nectarines, sweet potatoes, tomatoes, pumpkin, squash, lettuce, and most other vegetables and fruits serve as sources of β-carotene and other provitamin A carotenoids.

Evaluation of nutritional status

The most common procedure to evaluate vitamin A status is to measure the retinol level in plasma or serum. The normal range of vitamin A content for a child is 20 to 90 μg/dl; for an adult, the normal range is 30 to 90 μg/dl. Lower values are indicators of deficiency or depleted body stores. Serum values greater than 100 μg/dl are indicative of toxic levels of vitamin A. Retinol esters may also be observed in fasting blood with the intake of toxic quantities of the vitamin.

Vitamin A (continued)

Dark adaptation tests and electroretinogram measurements are also useful but difficult to perform on young children. Measurements of plasma retinol–binding protein levels can also serve as an indication of vitamin A nutritional status because they correlate with plasma retinol levels.

Signs, symptoms, and treatment of deficiency state

Skin lesions, such as follicular hyperkeratosis (Fig. 6-1), and night blindness are among the earliest signs of vitamin A deficiency. Severe depletion may result in conjunctival xerosis (drying) and progress to corneal ulceration, perforation, and finally destruction of the eye (keratomalacia). These changes are usually seen in children. Rapidly proliferating tissues are sensitive to vitamin A deficiency and may revert to an undifferentiated state. The bronchorespiratory tract, skin, genitourinary system, gastrointestinal tract, and sweat glands are adversely affected.

In cases of severe vitamin A deficiency in children, a single intramuscular injection of 30 mg of retinol (as palmitate) has been used. The World Health Organization treatment for vitamin A deficiency in children older than 1 year is the use of 110 mg of retinol palmitate orally or 55 mg intramuscularly, plus another 110 mg orally the following day and again prior to discharge.

Use and effects of large doses

An intake of retinoids greatly in excess of requirements results in a toxic condition known as hypervitaminosis A. It may occur in children as well as adults because of overzealous prophylactic vitamin therapy, extended self-medication, food fads, or use of high doses for the therapy of acne or other skin lesions. A daily intake of more than 7.5 mg (about 37,000 IU) of retinol is not advised, and chronic use of amounts over 20 mg (100,000 IU) can result in dry and itching skin, desquamation, erythematous dermatitis, hair loss, joint pain, chapped lips, hyperostosis (bony deposits), headaches, anorexia, edema, and fatigue. Vitamin A has been helpful in the treatment of certain skin diseases. Retinoids such as tretinoin (for acne) and isotretinoin (for recalcitrant cystic acne) have largely replaced the use of retinol for these conditions.

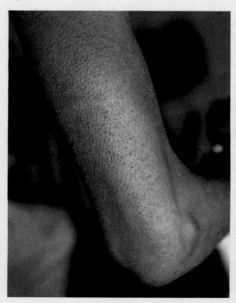

Fig. 6-1 Follicular hyperkeratosis in vitamin A deficiency.

Vitamin B₆

Physiology and biochemical pathways

Vitamin B₆ comprises the compounds pyridoxine, pyridoxal, and pyridoxamine. The three forms can interconvert in the body. Vitamin B₆ in the phosphorylated coenzyme form takes part in numerous reactions mostly associated with protein metabolism. The reactions include transanimations, deamination, and decarboxylation. The functions of vitamin B₆ are diverse and include glycine and serine interconversion; homocystine conversion to cystathionine; niacin and serotonin formation from tryptophan; and formation of δ-aminolevulinic acid for heme synthesis. The vitamin is present in phosphorylase, the enzyme which converts glycogen to glucose-1-phosphate.

Absorption

Most of the phosphorylated forms of vitamin B₆ are hydrolyzed by intestinal phosphates before absorption. Vitamin B₆ is absorbed by a nonsaturable process. Vitamin B₆ from some plant products may be present in bound forms (β-glucoside conjugates) that are not biologically available for the human.

Metabolism and excretion

The liver plays a major role in the conversion of pyridoxine to pyridoxal and pyridoxal phosphate for use by other tissues. With cirrhosis, the hepatic levels of vitamin B₆ are considerably reduced, and the ability to convert pyridoxine to pyridoxal phosphate is impaired. Pyridoxal phosphate is the main form of vitamin B₆ in plasma. The phosphorylated forms of vitamin B₆ are tightly bound to albumin and unavailable to tissues. Free pyridoxal is readily taken up by tissues. Small amounts of vitamin B₆ are excreted into the urine. The majority of ingested vitamin B₆ is converted to 4-pyridoxic acid and excreted. Stores of vitamin B₆ in the body are small (20 to 30 mg) and can be depleted within 30 days with the ingestion of vitamin B₆–deficient diets.

Recommended dietary allowance and nutrient interactions

The requirement for vitamin B₆ increases with the amount of protein in the diet. With an average intake of 100 g of protein per day, 2.2 mg of pyridoxine per day is required by adults. Lower intakes of protein may reduce the need for vitamin B₆ to 1.5 mg per day. Some women using oral contraceptives may have an increased requirement for vitamin B₆. In general, this effect is of minor clinical concern. Prolonged use of drugs such as isoniazid, penicillamine, cycloserine, and hydralazine may require vitamin B₆ supplements to reduce the neurological side effects. Vitamin B₆ supplements in patients receiving levodopa for the treatment of Parkinson's disease should be avoided.

Food sources

The majority of vitamin B₆ is present in food in the form of pyridoxine, pyridoxal phosphate, and pyridoxamine phosphate. Vitamin B₆ losses are often high in the processing and canning of meats and vegetables and in the milling of wheat. Fish, poultry, and other meats are good sources of the vitamin, as are vegetables such as carrots, cabbage, peas, potatoes, tomatoes, brussels sprouts, and cauliflower.

Evaluation of nutritional status

Vitamin B₆ status may be evaluated with the use of several laboratory procedures. Blood transaminase activities and xanthurenic acid excretion following a tryptophan load are commonly used for assessment. Plasma levels of pyridoxal and pyridoxal phosphate or the urinary excretion of 4-pryridoxic acid are also useful indices.

Signs, symptoms, and treatment of deficiency state

Vitamin B₆ deficiency is rarely encountered, and the clinical signs and symptoms associated with deficiency are not well established. The most common clinical manifestations associated with vitamin B₆ deficiency are central nervous system changes and abnormal

Vitamin B$_6$ (continued)

electroencephalograms. Hyperirritability and convulsive seizures may occur in infants. In adults, one is more likely to see eczema and seborrheic dermatitis in the regions of the ears, nose, and mouth; chapped lips; glossitis; and angular stomatitis. Occasionally, hypochromic, microcytic anemia may be observed. Increased excretion of xanthurenic acid occurs because of impaired metabolism of tryptophan with vitamin B$_6$ deficiency. Since a deficiency of vitamin B$_6$ would probably be associated with deficiencies of one or more other B vitamins, treatment with a B-complex multivitamin preparation is appropriate. In the United States, symptoms of B$_6$ deficiency are most likely to be seen in the form of neuritis due to isoniazid treatment.

Use and effects of large doses

Vitamin B$_6$-dependent syndromes will require treatment with high doses of the vitamin. Pyridoxine has low toxicity. However, daily supplements of 200 mg of pyridoxine over several months may result in a dependency when the supplement is discontinued. A toxic sensory neuropathy has been reported in people consuming more than 500 mg daily for an extended period. Isoniazid combines with pyridoxal or pyridoxal phosphate to inactivate the vitamin. Supplements of pyridoxine may be necessary to compensate for this inactivation. Vitamin B$_6$ reduces the beneficial effects of levodopa in the treatment of Parkinson's disease.

Vitamin B_{12}

Physiology and biochemical pathways

Vitamin B_{12} is a generic term for cobalamins that are active in humans. Structurally, vitamin B_{12} contains cobalt and a corrin moiety. Two cobalamins, 5′,-deoxyadenosyl-cobalamin and methylcobalamin, function as vitamin B_{12} coenzymes in humans. Vitamin B_{12} is also commonly called *cyanocobalamin*. Deoxyadenosylcobalamin is a cofactor of the mitochondrial mutase enzyme that catalyzes the isomerization of methylmalonyl coenzyme A to succinyl coenzyme A, an essential reaction in lipid and carbohydrate metabolism. Methylcobalamin is essential in folate metabolism because of its participation in the methionine synthetase reaction. The interaction of the two vitamins is essential for the conversion of homocysteine to methionine, for protein biosynthesis, for synthesis of purines and pyrimidines, for methylation reactions, and for the maintenance of intracellular levels of folates.

Absorption

Impaired absorption of vitamin B_{12} is most commonly associated with pernicious anemia, wherein the patient usually has a deficiency in the production of gastric intrinsic factor essential for the absorption of the vitamin (see Chapter 2). Intrinsic factor is a highly specific binding glycoprotein secreted by parietal cells of the stomach. In the normal person, vitamin B_{12} is absorbed through receptor sites in the distal ileum. Transcobalamin II, present in the plasma, transports vitamin B_{12} to the tissues that require it.

Metabolism and excretion

Various diseases and complications can interfere with the absorption of vitamin B_{12}. Included are gastric achlorhydria and decreased secretion of intrinsic factor secondary to gastric atrophy (such as with aging and pernicious anemia) or total gastrectomy; impaired pancreatic function accompanied by reduced production of proteins necessary for the release of vitamin B_{12} from proteins; production of antibodies to intrinsic factor; and damage by disease to ileal mucosal cells or surgical removal of the distal ileum. In vitamin B_{12} deficiency, folate becomes trapped as methyltetrahydrofolate to produce a deficiency in functional folate essential for hematopoiesis and other reactions. Vitamin B_{12} is stored in the hepatic parenchymal cells, where 1 to 10 mg may be present, representing up to 90% of the body's store of the vitamin. About 3 μg of vitamin B_{12} are secreted into the bile each day but are normally reabsorbed in the ileum. Little of the vitamin appears in the urine.

Recommended dietary allowance and nutrient interactions

Studies involving body stores and turnover rates of vitamin B_{12} indicate that 0.1% to 0.2% of the vitamin is lost from the body daily. Based on these investigations, the Recommended Daily Allowance (RDA) for vitamin B_{12} for adults is 2 μg/day, which allows for incomplete absorption and provides for a substantial body reserve. For the infant, an intake of 0.5 μg/day is recommended. During pregnancy and lactation, an additional intake of 2.2 μg/day is recommended (see Table 1-1).

Food sources

Microorganisms are the sole source of vitamin B_{12} in nature. All plants are devoid of vitamin B_{12}. Consequently, strict vegetarian diets are free of vitamin B_{12}. Animal products, including meats and meat products (especially liver, kidney, and heart), fish, poultry, shellfish, eggs, milk, and dairy products are the usual dietary sources. Vitamin B_{12} is rather stable to heat and usual cooking practices.

Evaluation of nutritional status

Measurement of serum vitamin B_{12} levels is commonly used to evaluate vitamin B_{12} status. Radioassays or microbiological assays are available for the determination. Serum levels

Vitamin B$_{12}$ (continued)

below 200 pg/ml indicate low body stores of vitamin B$_{12}$. Levels below 100 pg/ml are generally diagnostic of a vitamin B$_{12}$ deficiency. Red-cell vitamin B$_{12}$ levels are less reliable than serum levels for evaluating vitamin B$_{12}$ status.

Methylmalonate excretion associated with vitamin B$_{12}$ deficiency is seldom measured as an index of vitamin B$_{12}$ status. The deoxyuridine suppression test is useful in the assessment of vitamin B$_{12}$ nutriture, but the test is not simple to perform.

Signs, symptoms, and treatment of deficiency state

Deficiency of vitamin B$_{12}$ will result in a sore tongue, paresthesias of the extremities (numbness and tingling), weakness, and other neurologic changes. Vitamin B$_{12}$ deficiency can also cause megaloblastic anemia. Prolonged deficiency can result in irreversible damage to the nervous system. A deficiency of either vitamin B$_{12}$ or folate will result in a morphologically identical macrocytic anemia, megaloblastic bone marrow changes, and hypersegmented polymorphonuclear neutrophils (Fig. 2-6A). Because of the close metabolic relationship between vitamin B$_{12}$ and folate, vitamin B$_{12}$ nutritional status must also be evaluated in terms of folacin nutrition before therapy is initiated. When a dietary deficiency of vitamin B$_{12}$ occurs (as with vegans), an oral supplement of 1 μg/day is adequate. When the deficiency is due to inadequate absorption, monthly injections of 100 μg are adequate therapy or oral therapy of 1000 μg/day. Such patients should have their serum vitamin B$_{12}$ levels monitored every 6 to 12 months.

Use and effects of large doses

Vitamin B$_{12}$ has very low toxicity. However, the use of megadoses of the vitamin has application only in the treatment of the rare situation in which there is a congenital defect in vitamin B$_{12}$ metabolism (i.e., vitamin B$_{12}$-responsive methylmalonic acidemia).

Vitamin C (Ascorbic Acid)

Physiology and biochemical pathways

Vitamin C exists in two forms, ascorbic acid and dehydroascorbic acid, although most of the vitamin exists as ascorbic acid. Specific biochemical functions of vitamin C are incompletely defined, but it appears to participate in a number of reactions, mostly involving oxidation. As such, vitamin C participates in the hydroxylation of proline to hydroxyproline and lysine to hydroxylysine. Consequently, impairment of collagen synthesis occurs in vitamin C deficiency. Vitamin C also participates in the synthesis of carnitine, tyrosine, adrenal hormones, and vasoactive amines and in microsomal drug metabolism, leukocyte functions, folate metabolism, and wound healing.

Absorption

Absorption of vitamin C appears to occur in the distal region of the small intestine by means of a sodium-dependent active transport system. Some ascorbic acid may also be absorbed at a slow rate by simple diffusion. Normally 80% to 90% of dietary intake of vitamin C (up to 100 mg/day) is absorbed. Higher intake is less well absorbed.

Metabolism and excretion

Absorbed vitamin C readily equilibrates throughout the body pool. The average adult has a body pool of between 1.2 and 2 g that is used at a rate of 3% to 4% per day. Highest concentrations of the vitamin are found in the adrenal and pituitary glands, with lesser amounts in the brain, liver, pancreas, and spleen. Daily intake of 60 mg of vitamin C will provide for a body pool of approximately 1.5 g of the vitamin. Excess vitamin C is readily excreted in the urine as metabolites or unchanged ascorbic acid. The renal threshold for ascorbic acid is about 1.5 mg/dl of plasma.

Recommended dietary allowance and nutrient interaction

An interaction appears to exist between vitamin C, iron, and copper that influences normal heme function through the oxidation-reduction of iron and/or by regulating iron absorption and availability at the intestinal level. The absorption of nonheme iron in the diet can be enhanced fourfold or more by the simultaneous ingestion of 25 to 75 mg of vitamin C. The RDA for vitamin C is given in Table 1-1. The vitamin C requirement of cigarette smokers is higher than that of nonsmokers by as much as 50%. The use of oral contraceptives lowers the plasma concentrations of ascorbic acid; however, the significance of this observation is not known. Studies suggest that the elderly may have an increased requirement for vitamin C. Working in a hot environment also may increase the requirement for the vitamin.

Food sources

Vitamin C is highly water soluble but is labile in solution and readily destroyed by heat, oxidation, and alkali. Relatively large amounts of the vitamin are present in most fruits, including strawberries, citrus fruits, and tomatoes, and in various vegetables, including green peppers, broccoli, cauliflower, cabbage, and greens.

Evaluation of nutritional status

The measurement of serum or plasma levels of ascorbic acid is the most commonly used and practical procedure for evaluating vitamin C status. Serum vitamin C levels of 0.2 to 0.3 mg/dl indicate low or inadequate intake of the vitamin. Levels below 0.2 mg/dl indicate deficiency. Leukocyte vitamin C levels can provide information concerning body stores of the vitamin, but the analytical measurement is somewhat tedious.

Signs, symptoms, and treatment of deficiency

A deficiency of vitamin C can lead to scurvy. Scurvy is associated with a defect in collagen synthesis that is demonstrated by impacted hair follicles, corkscrew hairs, failure of wounds to heal, defects in tooth formation, and rupture of capillaries that leads to

Vitamin C (Ascorbic Acid) (continued)

perifollicular petechiae—pinpoint hemorrhages—and ecchymoses—large areas of dermal hemorrhage (Figs. 6-2A and B). Scurvy may be associated with loosening of the teeth (see Fig. 2-5), gingivitis, and anemia. Adults with scurvy should be given 1 g of ascorbic acid daily.

Use and effects of large doses

In the absence of scurvy, the administration of ascorbic acid in large amounts produces few demonstrable effects. Although megadoses of vitamin C have been reported to have beneficial effects on the common cold and to increase resistance to various diseases, these claims have not been well documented or accepted. For most individuals, ascorbic acid has low toxicity, and excessive intake is tolerated. Adverse effects include diarrhea, increased uric acid excretion, and hemolysis in patients with erythrocyte glucose–6-phosphate dehydrogenase deficiency. Large doses may interfere with tests for glucose in the urine (false-negative with the glucose-oxidase method, false-positive with copper reagents), may give a false-negative result in tests for occult blood in the stool, and may interfere with anticoagulant (heparin and coumadin) therapy.

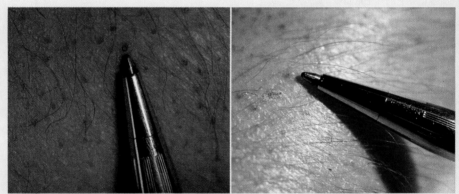

A

B

Fig. 6-2 **A,** Corkscrew hairs in scurvy. **B,** Perifollicular petechiae in scurvy.

Vitamin D
Physiology and biochemical pathways
The intestinal absorption of calcium and phosphorus is stimulated by the active metabolic of vitamin D, 1,25-dihydroxycholecalciferol (1,25-$(OH)_2D_3$), and as such, vitamin D serves as a regulator of calcium and phosphorus homeostasis. Vitamin D occurs in two forms: vitamin D_2 (ergocalciferol) and vitamin D_3 (cholecalciferol). Vitamin D_3 is the naturally occurring form and is produced by the action of sunlight on the 7-dehydrocholesterol in the skin. Vitamin D_2 is formed by ultraviolet irradiation of the plant sterol ergosterol. Vitamin D_2 and vitamin D_3 appear to be equally active in humans. Vitamin D is required for maintenance of skeletal integrity and proper utilization of calcium and phosphorus. Infants and children have the greatest need for vitamin D. When intake is inadequate, rickets may develop. In adults, osteomalacia may occur as a result of vitamin D deficiency.

Absorption
Dietary vitamin D is absorbed from the duodenum and jejunum in association with fat and is incorporated primarily into chylomicrons that are taken up by the liver. Fat malabsorption impairs the absorption of vitamin D.

Metabolism and excretion
Cholecalciferol is hydroxylated in the liver to produce 25-OH-D_3. The most potent metabolite of vitamin D, 1,25-$(OH)_2D_3$, is produced in the kidneys and is controlled according to requirements for growth, pregnancy, and lactation. Its formation is stimulated by parathyroid hormone, low serum phosphate, estrogen, prolactin, and growth hormone, and it appears to decrease with aging. Vitamin D is degraded by hepatic hydroxylases and excreted in the bile. Only 2% is excreted in the urine.

Recommended dietary allowance and nutrient interactions
Vitamin D requirements are expressed in terms of micrograms of cholecalciferol or in international units; 1 μg of cholecalciferol is equal to 40 IU. The RDA for vitamin D is shown in Table 1-1.

Food sources
The need for vitamin D is normally met by the action of sunlight on 7-dehydrocholesterol in the skin to produce vitamin D_3. In areas where sunlight is limited seasonally, the formation of vitamin D may be inadequate to meet needs. The sources of dietary vitamin D are limited primarily to liver, eggs, butter, fortified milk, and fatty fish.

Evaluation of nutritional status
Vitamin D nutritional status may be evaluated through the measurement of serum levels of 25-OH-D_3 and of 1,25-$(OH)_2D_3$. Serum measurements of 25-OH-D_3 provide a reliable index of vitamin D stores. Levels of 1,25-$(OH)_2D_3$ are less reliable for this purpose. For adults, an acceptable level of serum 25-OH-D_3 is 20 ng/ml, while serum 1,25-$(OH)_2D_3$ is 20 to 40 pg/ml. Vitamin D deficiency may be accompanied by a decrease in serum phosphate and calcium and an increase in serum alkaline phosphatase, urinary hydroxyproline, and parathyroid hormone levels. Roentgenogram findings may assist in the evaluation of rickets and osteomalacia.

Signs, symptoms, and treatment of deficiency state
Both rickets and osteomalacia are not commonly seen in the United States. Rickets in children is characterized by disorders of cartilage cell growth, enlargement of the epiphyseal growth plates, and accumulation of unmineralized bone matrix (Fig. 6-3). In adults, vitamin D deficiency causes osteomalacia. Patients receiving anticonvulsant agents (i.e., phenobarbital or phenytoin) for prolonged periods may develop rickets or osteomalacia.

Vitamin D (continued)

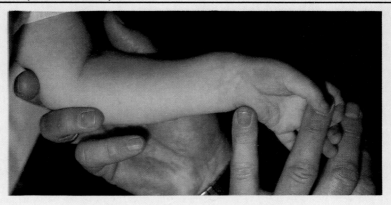

Fig. 6-3   Radial thickening seen in vitamin D deficiency.

Breast-fed infants or those fed unfortified formula should receive 400 units of vitamin D daily as a supplement. Fully developed rickets is often treated with 1,000 units of vitamin D daily. The major therapeutic uses of vitamin D are for prevention and cure of nutritional rickets, treatment of metabolic rickets and osteomalacia, and treatment of hypoparathyroidism. Chronic renal failure may be characterized by a decreased ability of the kidneys to convert 25-OH-D$_3$ to 1,25-(OH)$_2$D$_3$.

Use and effects of large doses

Toxicity caused by excess vitamin D administration is associated with plasma 25-OH-D$_3$ concentrations of more than 400 ng/ml. The initial signs and symptoms of vitamin D toxicity are weakness, fatigue, headache, nausea, vomiting, hypercalcemia, and impaired renal function. Hypercalcemia may arrest growth in children. Large doses of vitamin D cause bone decalcification. Because of the potential for toxicity, vitamin D should not be administered in excess of the RDA in Table 1-1.

Vitamin E

Physiology and biochemical pathways

Vitamin E is the name given to the family of tocopherols with a substituted chromanol ring and a saturated or unsaturated side chain. The biological activity of these vitamins is proportional to their proficiency as antioxidants, with α-tocopherol having the highest activity. One international unit has been defined as 1 mg of dl-tocopheryl acetate, a synthetic form of the vitamin. Synthetic dl-tocopherol has a potency of 1.1 IU/mg. One international unit is equivalent to 0.67 mg of dietary α-tocopherol, although various forms of vitamin E have differing activities.

The vitamin is lipid soluble and is found in all cell membranes. The greatest amount is found in adipose tissue, where the concentration is approximately 1 mg/g of lipid. The biological function of vitamin E is not specific in the sense that it participates as a coenzyme for enzyme-catalyzed reactions. The role of vitamin E as a free radical scavenger appears to be its primary biological function. In this capacity it scavenges free radicals generated by oxidases (i.e., xanthine oxidase and cytochrome P450–dependent oxidases) and generated by the breakdown of hydrogen peroxide. In this process the chromanol ring is converted to the relatively stable free radical tocopheroxyl, which may react with oxygen to form quinone. In the absence of the vitamin, free radicals peroxidize and oxidize polyunsaturated fatty acids resulting in membrane dysfunction, altered lipoprotein metabolism, and the deposition of lipofuscin or ceroid pigment (granules composed of oxidized lipid and protein).

Absorption

Vitamin E is absorbed in the proximal small intestine through a process that requires bile and pancreatic enzymes. Absorption is impaired in chronic cholestasis and pancreatic insufficiency. Transport from the intestine is via chylomicrons and is similar to that of dietary triglyceride. Thus, abetalipoproteinemia impairs transport.

Metabolism and excretion

Tocopherols protect polyunsaturated fatty acids in cellular and intracellular membranes from peroxidative damage. Thus the function of tocopherol is complementary to the function of glutathione peroxidase (a selenoenzyme), which catalyzes the reduction (i.e., detoxification) of peroxides in the cytoplasm.

Oxidation of tocopherol to quinone destroys the biological activity of the vitamin. Quinone and other oxidized metabolites are found in urine and feces. Ascorbic acid may reduce the tocopheroxyl radical or tocopherones (another oxidation product) back to tocopherol and may recycle the vitamin.

Recommended dietary allowance and nutrient interactions

The RDA for vitamin E varies with age, sex, pregnancy, and lactation. Recommended amounts are listed in Table 1-1. Requirements may be increased by the intake of foods high in polyunsaturated fatty acids and low in the vitamin (e.g., fish oil). Large doses of vitamin E interfere with vitamin K metabolism and should be avoided during anti-coagulant therapy. Doses of 400 mg/day of α-tocopherol also interfere with arachidonic-acid metabolism. Vitamin E absorption by infants is poor, and there is some evidence that low–birth weight and premature infants need at least 8 mg of tocopherol per day. Oxidation of polyunsaturated fatty acids (as measured by breath pentane) in smokers has been reduced by supplements of 800 mg/day.

Food sources

As a rule, tocopherols are present in vegetable oils in proportion to the linoleic acid content of the triglyceride. Therefore, good sources of the vitamin include cottonseed, corn, soybean, and safflower oil. Other moderately good sources include yellow-green vegetables, eggs, and whole-grain food products.

Vitamin E (continued)

Evaluation of nutritional status

There are high-performance liquid chromatography (HPLC) and colorimetric assays for serum and plasma vitamin E. Normal values are 0.5 to 1.2 mg/dl. Greater than 10% hemolysis by the peroxide-induced erthrocyte hemolysis test is also an indication of deficiency, because this value corresponds to a vitamin E concentration of approximately 0.4 mg/dl. A substantial number of children younger than 12 years of age may have serum levels below 0.5 mg/dl but have normal peroxide-induced erythrocyte hemolysis tests. Vitamin E mobilized from liver is bound to very low–density lipoproteins; therefore, hypoplipidemic patients will have lower serum levels. There is some evidence that a ratio of serum tocopherol to total lipid is a better indicator of nutriture. A value below 0.8 mg tocopherol/g of total serum lipid is considered deficient in adults and children.

Signs, symptoms, and treatment of deficiency

The cell membranes of a variety of organs may be altered by vitamin E deficiency; therefore, signs and symptoms may be nonspecific. Signs and symptoms include hemolytic anemia, myopathy with creatinuria, weakness, ataxia, impaired reflexes, ophthalmoplegia, retinopathy, and bronchopulmonary dysplasia (if on a respirator). In severe deficiency, permanent damage to nerve tissue has been demonstrated while psychomotor dysfunction has been demonstrated in some vitamin E–deficient patients. However, pure dietary deficiency is rare. Premature and low-birth-weight infants and patients with cholestasis and other fat malabsorption syndromes are predisposed to vitamin E deficiency. Deficiency states may be corrected with oral intake of 0.2 to 2 g. In the case of severe malabsorption, the parenteral route may be used.

Use and effects of large doses

Large doses of vitamin E have been used prophylactically in premature infants to protect against hemolytic anemia, retinopathy, and bronchopulmonary dysplasia. Large doses are also indicated in chronic cholestasis, pancreatic insufficiency, uncontrolled celiac disease, and other fat malabsorption syndromes. In addition, certain rare inborn errors of metabolism that result in hemolytic anemia also respond. These include glucose–6-phosphate dehydrogenase deficiency, thalassemia major, glutathione peroxidase deficiency, and glutathione synthesis deficiency. Treatment of sickle cell anemia also has been tried.

Vitamin E, unlike other fat-soluble vitamins, is remarkably nontoxic. High doses may interfere with vitamin K metabolism, resulting in an increase of clotting time, and may interfere with arachidonic acid and prostaglandin metabolism. Impaired immune function, increased sepsis, and impaired wound healing have been reported in infants treated with high doses. On the other hand, ingestion of up to 500 mg/day for 3 years failed to produce evidence of toxicity.

Vitamin K

Physiology and biochemical pathways

A vitamin K–dependent process in the liver is responsible for the synthesis of prothrombin (factor II), the zymogen of the blood coagulation enzyme thrombin. In the absence of vitamin K or in the presence of vitamin K antagonists such as sodium warfarin, vitamin K–dependent posttranslational glutamyl carboxylase is inhibited, and abnormal forms of prothrombin are produced. These abnormal forms lack a full complement of γ-carboxyglutamic acid residues and are unable to bind calcium normally; thus, they are inactive in blood coagulation. The precise mechanism by which vitamin K activates the glutamyl γ-carboxylase is unclear. Vitamin K–dependent carboxylase activity is necessary for the formation of a number of proteins that contain δ-carboxyglutamic acid (GLA) residues. Included are clotting factors VII, IX, and X; osteocalcin; protein S; and protein C (Fig. 6-4).

Absorption

Vitamin K is absorbed from the diet in the small intestine by an apparent saturable, energy-dependent system and is incorporated into chylomicrons. Fat malabsorption syndromes are associated with reduced vitamin K absorption.

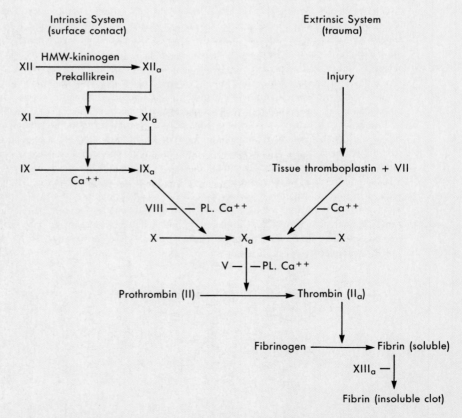

Fig. 6-4 The clotting cascade. (From Shils ME, Young VR: *Modern Nutrition in Health and Disease*, ed 7, Philadelphia, Lea & Febiger, 1988.)

Vitamin K (continued)

Metabolism and excretion

No specific plasma carrier has been identified for vitamin K. It is distributed to tissues via low-density lipoproteins. Vitamin K is present in tissues in only small amounts, with very little long-term storage. Vitamin K localizes in various cellular membranes, particularly in the golgi and smooth microsomal membrane fractions. Vitamin K_1 is rapidly metabolized to more polar metabolites and excreted in the urine and bile.

Recommended dietary allowance and nutrient interactions

A specific recommended allowance for vitamin K has not been established because of the variable contribution from the synthesis of the vitamin K forms by the intestinal flora. For adults, a daily intake of 65 to 80 µg is suggested; for infants, a daily intake of 10 µg is suggested. Mature breast milk provides approximately 15 µg of vitamin K per liter. Infant formulas usually contain a minimum of 4 µg of vitamin K per 100 kcal.

Food sources

Vitamin K is a fat-soluble compound that occurs naturally in two forms: vitamin K_1 (phylloquinone), which is present in green plants, and vitamin K_2 (menaquinones), produced by microorganisms. Green leafy vegetables are good sources of vitamin K_1, with lesser amounts provided by cereals, fruits, dairy products, and meats. The average diet is estimated to provide 300 to 500 µg of vitamin K_1 daily.

Evaluation of nutritional status

The adequacy of vitamin K intake is commonly evaluated by measuring the plasma concentration of one of the vitamin K–dependent clotting factors: prothrombin (factor II), factor VII, factor IX, or factor X. In the clinical laboratory, the one-stage prothrombin-time (PT) measurement is the standard procedure used to determine the extrinsic-pathway clotting time. Methods are available to measure the specific clotting factors but are generally not used to monitor vitamin K adequacy.

Signs, symptoms, and treatment of deficiency state

Uncomplicated cases of dietary inadequacy of vitamin K seldom occur, because the vitamin can be synthesized by intestinal flora. However, excess intake of large amounts of vitamin E can antagonize the action of vitamin K. Certain drug therapies such as warfarin, phenytoin, sulfa drugs, neomycin, and salicylates may interfere with vitamin K metabolism. The only known symptom of vitamin K deficiency in humans is increased prothrombin time, often associated with easy bruisability (Fig. 6-5).

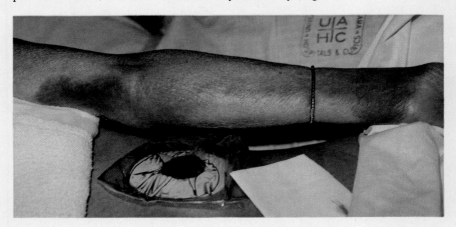

Fig. 6-5   Easy bruisability in vitamin K deficiency.

Vitamin K (continued)

Vitamin K deficiency occurs most commonly in newborns. Vitamin K does not cross the placental membrane well; thus, tissue stores are low in the newborn. Newborns also lack the intestinal flora necessary to synthesize vitamin K. A single dose of 0.5 to 1 mg of vitamin K is routinely parenterally administered to newborn infants.

In fat malabsorption syndromes, vitamin K deficiency may occur, especially if there is use of antibiotics that suppress the flora in the large bowel.

Use and effect of large doses

Patients with parenchymal liver disease may have hypothrombinemia because of an inability to utilize vitamin K in the biosynthesis of vitamin K–dependent clotting factors. Some patients respond favorably to a parenteral dose of 10 mg of vitamin K daily for 3 days. Vitamin K^1 (phylloquinone, phytonadione) is relatively nontoxic in humans, although rapid intravenous administration of vitamin K_1 has produced dyspnea, flushing, chest pains, cardiovascular collapse, and rarely, death. These effects may have been related to the dispersing agents rather than to the vitamin.

Excessive bleeding produced by administration of oral vitamin K antagonist anticoagulants, such as warfarin, can be corrected in a few hours by the administration of vitamin K_1 (phylloquinone). A single dose of 2.5 to 10 mg of vitamin K_1 has been used to treat a mild overdosage of anticoagulants (e.g., warfarin).

Biotin

Physiology and biochemical pathways

Biotin, a member of the vitamin B complex, is composed of fused tetrahydrothiophene and ureido rings with a valeric acid side chain. Covalent attachment to the apoenzyme forms the prosthetic group (biocytin). This is accomplished by the energy-dependent formation of an amide bond using the valeric acid side chain and the E amino group of a specific lysine residue in the apoenzyme. Biotin formation is catalyzed by the holoenzyme synthetase. Adenosine triphosphatase (ATP)-dependent carboxylation reactions are catalyzed by holoenzymes (e.g., acetyl-coenzyme A [CoA] propionyl-CoA, B-methyl-crotonyl-CoA, geranoyl-CoA, and pyruvate carboxylases), which are involved in fatty acid, cholesterol, protein, and carbohydrate metabolism. The central intermediate in these reactions is the N'carboxybiotinyl enzyme. Some storage of the vitamin occurs in the liver.

Absorption

Absorption of the vitamin occurs in the proximal small intestine by a sodium-dependent active transport mechanism. Biotin-synthesizing bacteria live in the intestine and contribute to body pools of available biotin. Clinical experiments have demonstrated that the vitamin is absorbed in the distal colon. Absorption of the vitamin from different foods varies considerably, although on average approximately 50% of dietary biotin is absorbed.

Metabolism and excretion

Normal activity of the holoenzyme synthetase and biotinidase (the enzyme that catalyzes the hydrolytic cleavage of biotin from the epsilon-amino group of lysine) is required for metabolism. It is therefore likely that turnover of the vitamin from one apoenzyme to another is required. Biotinidase also hydrolyzes lipoic acid from the epsilon-amino group of lysine. The principal excretory product is free intact biotin. Urinary and fecal excretion is greater than dietary intake, reflecting biosynthesis by gut flora.

Recommended dietary allowance and nutrient interactions

There is no RDA for biotin. The estimated safe and adequate daily intake is based approximately on 50 μg/1000 kcal and is shown in Table 1-1. Uncooked egg whites contain a glycoprotein, avidin, that binds the vitamin, making it unavailable for absorption.

Food sources

Good sources include liver, whole grain rice, and eggs. Other sources include nuts, cauliflower, cowpeas, mackerel, and sardines. Biotin occurs in the free form in plant-derived food and is bound to protein in animal-derived food. The average American diet includes 100 to 300 μg/day.

Evaluation of nutritional status

Microbiological and isotope dilution assays are most frequently used to evaluate the nutritional status of biotin. Whole blood levels and urinary levels are highly variable
Normal whole blood levels range from 200 to 500 pg/ml. Levels below 100 pg/ml may indicate deficiency. Normal urinary excretion ranges from 6 to more than 100 μg in 24 hours.

Signs, symptoms, and treatment of deficiency state

Biotin deficiency due to poor dietary intake is rare. Experimental biotin deficiency is characterized by dermatitis, hair loss (Figs. 6-6A and B), atrophy of the lingual papillae, graying of mucous membranes, muscle pain, paresthesias, hypercholesterolemia, and electrocardiogram abnormalities. Some of these signs and symptoms have been observed in people eating raw eggs and in patients given long-term, high-dose antibiotics. Total parenteral nutrition solutions used for long-term (>8 weeks) should contain biotin. Biotin deficiency responds to 300 μg/day for several days. Holoenzyme synthetase deficiency

Biotin (continued)

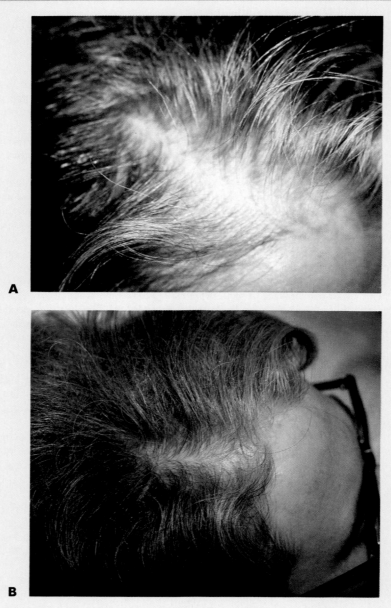

Fig. 6-6   Alopecia before **(A)** and after **(B)** biotin therapy in a patient on long-term total parenteral nutrition without biotin.

Biotin (continued)

is a rare inborn error of metabolism that is characterized by erythematous rash, persistent vomiting, and impaired immune function. The K_m for the enzyme is reported to be 500 times higher in these patients when compared with normal. The activity of all of the carboxylases is low.

Biotinidase deficiency also is a rare inborn error that results in delayed neuromotor development, nystagmus, hypotonia, impaired immune function, ketosis, and the accumulation of lactate in the tissues. In these patients, biotinidase activity in plasma is low; however, the activity of the carboxylases in normal.

Use and effects of large doses

Holoenzyme synthetase and biocytinase deficiency respond to 10 to 100 mg of biotin per day. Up to 10 mg/day over long periods of time has no toxicity in humans.

Folic Acid, Folate

Physiology and biochemical pathways

Folate describes a group of compounds that contain a pteridine ring, para-aminobenzoic acid and glutamic acid, and that possess the biological activity of folic acid (pteroylglutamic acid). Most natural folates are in polyglutamate forms containing additional glutamic acid residues bound in a peptide linkage. The folate polyglutamates are the functional coenzymes in tissues, where they participate primarily in one-carbon transfers. As such, they participate in purine and pyrimidine biosynthesis, formate metabolism, and amino acid interconversions (e.g., serine and glycine interconversions; homocysteine to methionine; histidine degradation to glutamic acid). Metabolic relationships exist between folate and vitamin B_{12}. A deficiency of either folate or vitamin B_{12} results in megaloblastic anemia as a result of impaired cell maturation and division.

Absorption

The presence of the different forms of folate in foods has resulted in uncertainties as to their bioavailability. On the average, 50% of dietary folate appears to be bioavailable. Before dietary folate can be absorbed, the polyglutamate forms must by hydrolyzed to monoglutamate forms by the conjugases present in the lumen and brush border of the intestine. Folate-binding proteins, associated with the brush border, appear to be involved in the transportation of folate across cell membranes. Part of the absorbed monoglutamate is converted to methyltetrahydrofolate and transferred into the portal circulation.

Malabsorption syndromes such as tropical sprue, celiac disease, and Crohn's disease adversely affect the absorption of folate. Impaired ability to absorb folate may occur in malnourished alcoholics and among users of certain drugs such as sulfasalazine.

Metabolism and excretion

5-Methyltetrahydrofolate is the predominant circulating form of folate. Pteroylglutamic acid (folic acid) is taken up by the liver and converted to 5-methyltetrahydrofolate, which is either stored in the liver (primarily in the polyglutamate form) or made available to the peripheral tissues. Alcoholic cirrhotics may have reduced retention of folate in the liver. The catabolism of folate is uncertain. Only small amounts of intact folate are excreted in the urine of normal individuals.

Recommended dietary allowance and nutrient interactions

The RDA for folate takes into account the bioavailability of dietary folate and an estimate of the amount required to maintain tissue stores of the vitamin. The recommended allowance for folate is given in Table 1-1.

Food sources

Folate is present in a wide variety of food items but is particularly plentiful in fresh green vegetables, liver, and some fresh fruits. As much as 50% to 95% of the folate present in foods may be lost during food processing and home cooking.

Evaluation of nutritional status

Measurement of folate levels in serum and red blood cells is the most practical and commonly used procedure to evaluate folate status. Measurements are provided by microbiological assay *(Lactobacillus casei)* or by radioassay. Plasma folate values above 6 ng/ml are considered acceptable, whereas values less than 3 ng/ml are considered deficient. Red blood cell folate levels above 160 ng/ml are considered acceptable, whereas values less than 140 ng/ml are considered deficient. Plasma folate reflects recent dietary intake, whereas red blood cell folate is an indicator of tissue stores. Some antibiotics and methotrexate may interfere with the microbiological assay. Histidine loading tests (formiminoglutamic acid excretion) and deoxyuridine suppression tests are not practical as routine indices of folate status. Patients with a suspected folate deficiency should be

Folic Acid, Folate (continued)

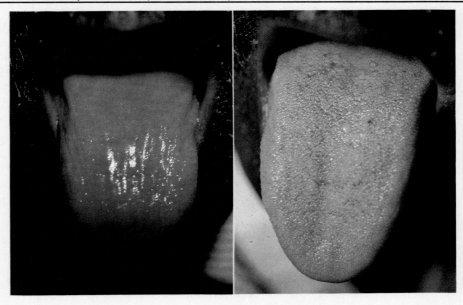

A   **B**

Fig. 6-7 Depapillation of the tongue. Slick tongue before (**A**) and after (**B**) folate replacement in an alcoholic patient.

evaluated further to eliminate the possibility of a coexisting biochemical vitamin B_{12} deficiency.

Signs, symptoms, and treatment of deficiency state

Folate deficiency results in megaloblastic anemia that cannot be distinguished from that caused by a deficiency of vitamin B_{12} (see Fig. 2-6). Folate deficiency rarely is associated with neurologic abnormalities that occur frequently with vitamin B_{12} deficiency. Severe folate deficiency may result in glossitis (Figs. 6-7A and B) and alterations in intestinal function due to abnormalities in the rapid turnover of the cells of the intestinal villi. Prior to treatment of megaloblastic anemia with folate, the absence of vitamin B_{12} deficiency must be established. Therapy with folate in the presence of vitamin B_{12} deficiency will correct the hematologic abnormalities but will not prevent progression of the neurologic defects associated with vitamin B_{12} deficiency. Pregnancy and lactation, with the increased demands, are situations in which folate supplementation of 400 µg/day of pteroylglutamic acid may be indicated. Patients with megaloblastic anemia should be evaluated to determine the effects of medications and alcohol intake. For folate-deficient adult patients, without sprue or intestinal malabsorption, an oral dose of 1 mg of folate/day is considered adequate. A supplement of 400 µg/day during pregnancy and 100 µg/day during lactation is suggested.

Use and effects of large doses

High doses of folate are used in limited instances. Oral dosages as high as 15 mg/day have been used for extended periods without side effects. However, large doses may counteract the antiepileptic effects of phenobarbital, primidone, and phenytoin. Leucovorin (5-formyl tetrahydrofolic acid), a metabolite of folate, is used to reverse the effects of antifolates such as methotrexate.

Vitamin B₃ (Niacin)

Physiology and biochemical pathways

Present in all cells, mainly in its amide form, nicotinamide is a structural component of the pyridine nucleotide coenzymes nicotinamide-adenine dinucleotide (NAD) and nicotinamide-adenine dinucleotide phosphate (NADP). Both coenzymes participate as cofactors in glycolysis and in many oxidation-reduction reactions or dehydrogenase systems central to tissue respiration. Tissues with high respiration rates, such as the central nervous system, are most extensively affected by niacin deficiency. Fatty acid synthesis requires NADPH, the reduced form of NADP, whereas oxidation of fatty acids requires NAD.

Humans are capable of converting tryptophan to niacin. Approximately 60 mg of tryptophan will provide 1 mg of niacin. Vitamin B₆ and riboflavin are essential for this conversion.

Absorption

Niacin is absorbed from the stomach and small intestine by a carrier-mediated, sodium-dependent facilitated diffusion process at low concentrations and by passive diffusion at higher concentrations. Absorption may be impaired as a result of chronic alcoholism. Niacin is present in animal foods largely as nicotinamide nucleotides with little free nicotinic acid or nicotinamide present. The nucleotides are converted to nicotinamide at the time of absorption.

Metabolism and excretion

Nicotinic acid is converted to nicotinamide by the nicotinamide dinucleotide pathway, but direct conversion has not been demonstrated. Nicotinamide is converted to N'methylnicotinamide, much of which is converted to N'-methyl-2-pyridone-5-carboxamide (2-pyridone). Normally, adults excrete 20% to 30% of their niacin as N'methylnicotinamide and 40% to 60% as the 2-pyridone. The amounts of intact niacin excreted in the urine are small and are influenced little by dietary intake of niacin or tryptophan.

Recommended dietary allowance and nutrient interactions

Allowance for niacin is expressed in terms of niacin equivalents, in which one niacin equivalent is equal to 1 mg of niacin or 60 mg of tryptophan. The RDA for niacin for adults is related to energy expenditure, in which 6.6 niacin equivalents are required per 1000 kcal. Additional allowances are made for pregnancy and lactation. (See Table 1-1.)

Food sources

Niacin is remarkably stable and can withstand considerable periods of cooking, storage, and heating. Legumes, cereals, and meats are good sources. However, niacin may be present in wheat, corn, and certain cereal products in bound forms (called niacytin) that are not biologically available to humans. Fish, poultry, and red meats with their high content of both niacin and tryptophan are excellent sources of niacin.

Evaluation of nutritional status

Laboratory procedures for the assessment of the nutritional status of this vitamin are limited. The only practical biochemical procedure is the measurement of the urinary levels of the niacin metabolites N'methylnicotinamide and 2-pyridone. The ratio of these values is used as an index of niacin nutritional status. Under normal conditions, a ratio of 1.4 to 4 exists between 2-pyridine and N'methylnicotinamide excretion. A ratio of less than 1 is indicative of niacin deficiency.

Signs, symptoms, and treatments of deficiency

Niacin deficiency results in pellagra, which is characterized by diarrhea, dermatitis, dementia, and ultimately death. Early symptoms may include anorexia, weakness, irritability, insomnia, glossitis, stomatitis, numbness, burning sensation in various parts of

Vitamin B₃ (Niacin) (continued)

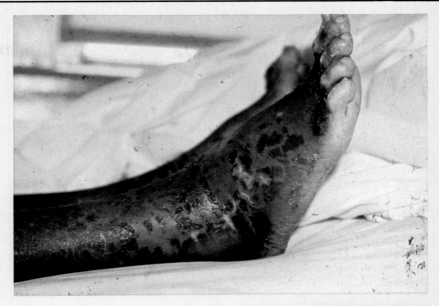

A

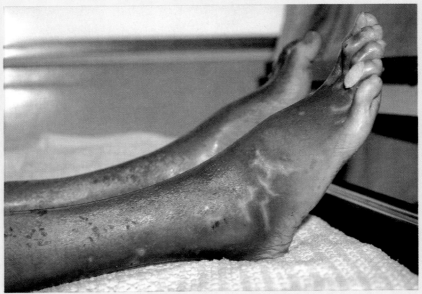

B

Fig. 6-8 Clinical findings of niacin deficiency before (**A**) and after (**B**) therapy in an alcoholic patient.

Vitamin B₃ (Niacin) (continued)

the body, vertigo, and forgetfulness. Intermittent constipation and diarrhea occur. The first lesions to appear are those of the mucous membranes of the mouth, tongue, and vagina. Pigmented keratotic scaling lesions are especially prominent on the areas of the body exposed to the sun, such as the face, hands, neck, feet, and forearms (Figs. 6-8A and B). Dementia is generally an advanced manifestation of the deficiency.

Treatment with either nicotinic acid or nicotinamide produces a prompt response, often within 24 hours. Nicotinamide is usually preferred in order to avoid the flushing reaction produced by nicotinic acid. Recommended treatment is an oral dose of 50 mg of niacin given up to 10 times daily or intravenous injections of 25 mg two or more times daily. Pellagra may occur in Hartnup disease because of impaired tryptophan utilization and in some patients with carcinoid tumors.

Use and effects of large doses

Nicotinic acid (but not nicotinamide) has been used as a vasodilator and to lower plasma cholesterol. Large doses of nicotinic acid may rapidly reduce plasma triglycerides and more slowly, plasma cholesterol. When used alone, triglycerides may be reduced by 20% to more than 80%, and plasma low-density lipoprotein (LDL) cholesterol often is reduced 10% to 15%. Used in combination with a bile acid–binding resin, a 40% to 60% reduction in plasma LDL cholesterol may be seen. High doses of nicotinic acid must be used with care because of adverse effects that may occur in patients, such as abnormalities in hepatic function, hyperglycemia, elevated plasma uric acid, and vasodilation.

Pantothenic Acid

Physiology and biochemical pathways

Pantothenic acid is a B-complex vitamin composed of a substituted butyric acid and β-alanine joined by a peptide bond. Pantothenic acid is a vitamin precursor of CoA and 4' phosphopantetheine, the prosthetic group of acyl carrier protein (ACP). More than 70 enzymes are known to require CoA or ACP. These enzymes are involved in fatty acid synthesis, lipid, carbohydrate, and amino acid metabolism, cholesterol synthesis, and many other pathways. Both CoA and ACP are required for acyl group transfer reaction; a thiol ester is the common intermediate.

Liver and adrenal glands have the highest concentration; however, body stores are small.

Absorption

Approximately 50% of the pantothenic acid in food is absorbed. Intestinal microflora may also be a source. Cellular uptake of pantothenate occurs by a specific saturable mechanism in concert with the cotransport of sodium ions.

Metabolism and excretion

Pantothenate is phosphorylated by ATP to yield 4'phosphopantetheine acid, followed by the addition and subsequent decarboxylation of cysteine to yield 4-phosphopantetheine. The addition of the elements of adenosine monophosphate (AMP) is followed by phosphorylation of ribose convert 4'phosphopantetheine to CoA. A phosphodiester is formed linking 4'phosphopantetheine to a serine of ACP. Urinary excretion of pantothenic acid is proportionate to intake. Normal urinary excretion is 2 to 7 mg/day; 1 to 2 mg/day is lost in feces.

Recommended dietary allowance and nutrient interactions

There is no RDA for pantothenic acid. Estimated safe and adequate daily intakes are listed in Table 1-2. Higher intakes may be required for pregnancy and lactation.

Food sources

Pantothenic acid is widely distributed in foods. Good sources include meats, whole grain cereals, and legumes.

Evaluation of nutritional status

Whole blood and urine pantothenate may be determined by microbiological assay and by radioimmunoassay following pantotheinase treatment of the specimen. Serum levels are considered unreliable as indicators of nutriture. Average whole blood levels are 100 to 300 μg/dl. Whole blood levels less than 100 μg/dl may indicate deficiency.

Signs, symptoms, and treatment of deficiency

There is little clinical evidence of dietary deficiency in humans. Experimentally, deficiency has been produced in subjects given ω-methylpantothenic acid (a metabolite antagonist) and in subjects consuming a semisynthetic diet deficient in the vitamin. Signs and symptoms include vomiting, malaise, abdominal distress, burning, cramps, fatigue, insomnia, and paresthesias of the hands and feet. Single, uncomplicated pantothenic acid deficiency is very rare. However, marginal deficiency may occur concurrent with other B-complex vitamin deficiencies.

Use and effects of large doses

Doses of up to 10 g/day have been given without toxicity. Diarrhea has been reported when doses of 10 to 20 g/day have been used.

Vitamin B₂ (Riboflavin)

Physiology and biochemical pathways

Riboflavin is a water-soluble B-complex vitamin and is composed of a substituted isoalloxazine ring and a ribitol side chain. The coenzyme forms of the vitamin—flavin mononucleotide (FMN) and flavin adenine dinucleotide (FAD)—bind reversibly to the apoenzyme; FAD binds covalently to succinic dehydrogenase, sarcosine dehydrogenase, and monoamine oxidase. Riboflavin-dependent enzymes catalyze a diverse array of chemical reactions, including one-electron transfers, pyridine and nonpyridine-dependent dehydrogenases, disulfide reductases, and oxygen and monoxygen reductases. These enzymes play an important role in amino acid metabolism, purine and pyrimidine metabolism, choline and fatty-acid oxidation, glycolysis, the tricarboxylic-acid cycle, and in the metabolism of vitamin K, folic acid, pyridoxamine, and niacin. The vitamin is not stored effectively. The coenzyme forms FMN and FAD found in food are hydrolyzed to riboflavin by nonspecific enzymes. Free riboflavin is found in milk and eggs.

Absorption

The major site of absorption of riboflavin is the proximal intestine. The process occurs via a saturable transport mechanism involving phosphorylation and dephosphorylation. The absorption process is saturated with 25 mg of the vitamin. Substantial amounts of circulating riboflavin are bound nonspecifically by serum albumin. Lesser amounts are bound by other plasma proteins.

Metabolism and excretion

Riboflavin is converted to FMN and FAD by the action of flavokinase and FAD pyrophosphorylase. It is likely that the biosynthesis of the apoenzyme occurs prior to covalent attachment of FAD. Both specific and nonspecific phosphatases hydrolyze FMN to riboflavin. Riboflavin is the major excretory product in urine and feces.

Recommended dietary allowance and nutrient interactions

The recommended allowance for riboflavin varies with age, sex, pregnancy, and lactation. The RDA is listed in Table 1-1. Riboflavin-dependent enzymes are involved in the biosynthesis of niacin from tryptophan and the transformation of coenzymes from pyridoxine, folic acid, and vitamin K.

Food sources

Good sources of riboflavin include milk, yogurt, cheese, meat, eggs, broccoli, asparagus, oranges, and whole-grain foods. The vitamin is unstable in light and heat.

Signs, symptoms, and treatment of deficiency

The signs and symptoms of riboflavin deficiency include nasolabial seborrheic dermatitis, cheilosis, glossitis, angular stomatitis (Figs. 6-9A and B), burning and itching of the eyes, corneal vascularization, and anemia.

Single uncomplicated riboflavin deficiency is rare, because food sources for other B-complex vitamins are the same and nutrient interactions complicate the clinical picture. Riboflavin metabolism is altered in patients treated with chlorpromazine, tetracycline, imipramine, amitriptyline, and phenothiazine. The evidence that the use of oral contraceptives increases requirements for riboflavin is controversial. However, alcoholism is a predisposing factor to alterations in riboflavin metabolism.

Riboflavin deficiency can usually be treated with an oral intake of 10 to 15 mg/day for 1 week. A parenteral preparation can be used when malabsorption is severe.

Evaluation of nutritional status

Erythrocyte glutathione reductase activity and stimulation by added FAD in vitro is the most common procedure. The upper limit of the normal range of stimulation is 76%. There are HPLC and spectrofluorimetric methods for detection in blood and urine. Also, egg white riboflavin–binding protein has been used to detect the vitamin in urine.

Vitamin B₂ (Riboflavin) (continued)

Use and effects of large doses

There are no reports of human toxicity. Toxicity in laboratory animals is very low. Three riboflavin-responsive inborn errors of metabolism have been reported. They include carnitine deficiency with lipid myopathy, short chain acyl-CoA dehydrogenase deficiency, and ethylmalonic-adipic aciduria.

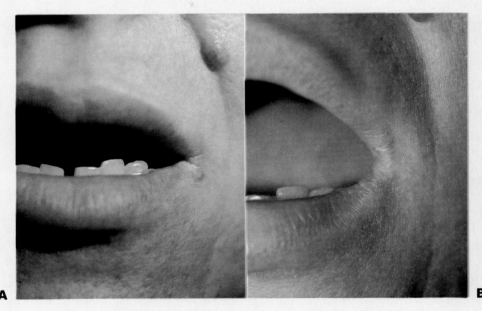

A   B

Fig. 6-9   Angular stomatitis of riboflavin deficiency before (A) and after (B) therapy.

Vitamin B₁ (Thiamin)

Physiology and biochemical pathways

Thiamin is a B-complex vitamin composed of a substituted pyrimidine and thiazole ring with a hydroxyethyl side chain. The coenzyme form of the vitamin, thiamin pyrophosphate (TPP), is required by enzymes involved in oxidative decarboxylation (e.g., pyruvate, ketoglutarate, and branched-chain keto acid decarboxylations) of glycolysis, tricarboxylic acid (TCA) cycle, and amino acid metabolism. TPP also is required by the transketolase enzyme in the pentose phosphate pathways.

Another important metabolic product of thiamin is thiamin triphosphate (TTP). TTP is thought to bind at or near the sodium channel in nerve membranes. Certain nerve toxins displace TTP from the nerve membrane in concert with blockage of the sodium channel. Dephosphorylation of TTP together with sodium influx may be required for nerve-impulse propagation.

Neither thiamin nor TPP is stored effectively. Clinical signs and symptoms of thiamin deficiency can appear in as little as 12 days if the diet is deficient.

Absorption

Absorption occurs in the upper small intestine by active transport at physiological concentrations and by passive diffusion at higher concentrations. Active thiamin transport may be coupled to a sodium-dependent phosphorylation of the vitamin. There is no binding protein in circulation.

Metabolism and excretion

Intracellularly, thiamin is converted to TPP by thiamin pyrophosphokinase. The most important organ for this reaction is the liver, because patients with cirrhosis have defective thiamin phosphorylation, and in these patients erythrocyte transketolase activity does not respond to thiamin therapy. TPP is the major form in the body, accounting for approximately 80% of the body pool; 50% of this is found in muscle. The high content in muscle probably reflects its demands for carbohydrate metabolism.

More than 20 metabolites of thiamin have been detected in human urine. In general, these metabolites are substituted pyrimidine-ring and thiazole-ring compounds. Alcohol dehydrogenase oxidizes the hydroxyethyl side chain of both thiamin and its thiazole moiety.

Recommended dietary allowance and nutrient interactions

The RDA for thiamin varies with age, sex, pregnancy, lactation, and energy intake. An intake of 0.5 mg of thiamin per 1000 kcal of energy is recommended with a minimum intake of 1 mg for adults. RDAs are found in Table 1-1.

Alcohol abuse and folate deficiency result in malabsorption of the vitamin. Vitamin antagonists include caffeic acid and tannic acid found in coffee and tea. Refeeding after starvation may precipitate the deficiency.

Food sources

Good food sources include lean pork, legumes, whole grain cereals, breads, and any enriched grain product.

Evaluation of nutritional status

The most common procedure for assessing thiamin status is the measurement of erythrocyte transketolase activity and its stimulation in vitro by added TPP. The upper limit of the normal range of stimulation is 23%; average normal stimulation is 12% to 15%. In patients with beriberi, average stimulation is 35%; in patients suffering from Wernicke's encephalopathy, the stimulation varies from 28% to 67%. Spectrofluorometric and HPLC methods are also used to determine thiamin levels in blood serum and urine. Average whole blood thiamin levels in control subjects are 68 ng/ml (ranges 50 to 80) and 39

Vitamin B₁ (Thiamin) (continued)

ng/ml in beriberi patients. Normal urinary excretion is greater than 60 μg/g creatinine in adults and greater than 150 μg/g creatinine in children.

Signs, symptoms, and treatment of deficiency

Classical thiamin deficiency, known as beriberi, is rare in this country, although alcoholics are at increased risk. Dry beriberi is characterized by chronic polyneuropathy with the following signs and symptoms: anorexia, ataxia, apathy, weakness, decreased attention span, calf tenderness, paresthesia, food drop (Fig. 6-10) and wrist drop, ophthalmoplegia (Fig. 6-11), and nystagmus. Wet beriberi is characterized by edema and high-output cardiac failure and may be rapidly precipitated by physical exercise or infection. Signs and symptoms include palpitations, shortness of breath, chest pain, increased systolic blood pressure, and pulmonary congestion. Neuropathy due to thiamin deficiency may be underdiagnosed in this country because of nonspecific symptoms such as weakness, leg cramping, and burning feet. Because beriberi is a medical emergency, aggressive treatment with 100 mg of intramuscular or intravenous thiamin hydrochloride daily is indicated. Response is usually noticeable in several hours. Treatment with other B-complex vitamins also is indicated.

Alcoholic polyneuropathy resulting from thiamin deficiency responds to 10 to 15 mg administered orally along with other B-complex vitamins.

Wernicke-Korsakoff syndrome may be an inborn error in metabolism resulting from a decreased affinity (high K_m of the transketolase enzyme for TPP) coupled with lower absolute levels of the transketolase. This syndrome is masked when the patient is thiamin replete and is unmasked by alcohol abuse, insufficient diet, or malabsorption. Some

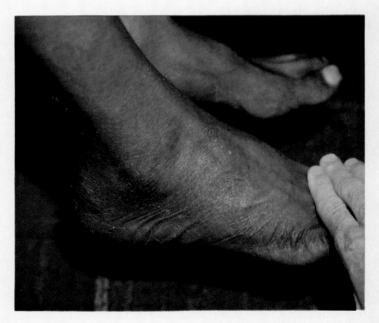

Fig. 6-10   Inability to dorsiflex the foot (foot-drop) in an alcoholic patient with thiamin deficiency.

Vitamin B₁ (Thiamin) (continued)

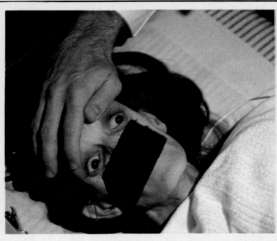

Fig. 6-11   Inability to follow a light source (ophthalmoplegia) due to thiamin deficiency and phosphorus deficiency.

characteristic signs and symptoms include ataxia, ophthalmoplegia, nystagmus, disorientation, severely impaired short-term memory, and confabulation. These patients usually respond to 100 mg administered intramuscularly or intravenously and to 10 to 15 mg/day of orally administered thiamin.

Use and effects of large doses

Thiamin-responsive inborn errors of metabolism (in addition to Wernicke-Korsakoff syndrome) include branched-chain keto-acid decarboxylase deficiency (maple syrup urine disease), pyruvate dehydrogenase deficiency (subacute necrotizing encephalomyelopathy), and megaloblastic anemia associated with diabetes mellitus. Oral dosages of 300 mg/day are nontoxic in humans; however, parenteral dosages greater than 400 mg/day may cause anorexia, lethargy, mild ataxia, and reduced tone of the intestinal tract.

7

Mineral and Trace Elements

Calcium
Iodine
Iron
Magnesium
Phosphorus
Zinc
Other trace elements

Calcium

Physiology and biochemical pathways

Calcium is the fifth most abundant element in the body, with 99% present in the bones. It is also the most abundant cation in the body. Calcium is required for the formation and maintenance of skeletal tissue and teeth and is essential for the functional integrity of nerve and muscle, where it influences excitability and muscle contraction and release of neurotransmitters. Blood clotting also is dependent upon calcium. Half of the plasma calcium is ionized and physiologically active and presumably under hormonal control. A significant decrease in plasma-ionized calcium will result in tetany and convulsions.

Absorption

Calcium is absorbed from the intestine by active transport. Vitamin D, as 1,25-dihydroxycholecalciferol ($1,25(OH)_2D_3$), is required for active calcium transport via the production of the vitamin D–dependent calcium-binding protein in the intestine. Some dietary factors enhance the absorption of calcium, such as certain amino acids (lysine and arginine) and lactose. High oxalate and phytate, present in some foods, may decrease calcium absorption. Unabsorbed fatty acids in the intestine (those present because of fat malabsorption due to intestinal diseases or resection of the small intestine) bind calcium, form unabsorbable compounds, and result in negative calcium balance.

Metabolism and excretion

The metabolism of calcium is controlled by parathyroid hormone, calcitonin, and vitamin D. Vitamin D stimulates intestinal absorption of calcium and decreases renal excretion. Calcium retention may be reduced by increased protein intake.

Recommended dietary allowance and nutrient interactions

Intake of large amounts of protein and sodium may increase calcium requirements. In the United States, the recommended intake of calcium is probably higher than in countries with lower usual intakes of protein-rich foods and salt. About 25% of adolescent American women and 50% of American women over 35 years of age consume less than 500 mg of calcium/day. The Recommended Daily Allowance (RDA) for calcium is shown in Table 1-1.

Food sources

Highly concentrated sources of calcium in the diet are cheeses, organ meats, egg yolks, sardines, almonds, collards, turnip greens, and mustard greens. Other good sources of calcium include shrimp, salmon, scallops, cereal grains, figs, other green vegetables, and dairy products such as milk, ice cream, and yogurt.

Evaluation of nutritional status

Suitable laboratory techniques for evaluating the adequacy of calcium intake do not exist. Serum calcium levels are closely controlled by the body over a wide range of intake. Low serum calcium values are more suggestive of a pathologic condition such as malabsorption syndrome, vitamin D deficiency, or hypoparathyroidism than of a dietary deficiency of calcium. Most cases of low serum calcium levels are a result of reduced circulating levels of albumin, because about 45% of serum calcium is albumin bound. Hypoalbuminemia decreases the serum total calcium by approximately 0.8 g/dl for each 1 g/dl decrease in albumin. In this situation, the active, ionizable fraction remains normal. Normal serum calcium levels range from 8.5 to 10.5 mg/dl (4.5 to 5.5 mEq/L). Bone roentgenograms, bone biopsy, and photon absorptiometry have been used to provide an indication of bone density and the existence of osteoporosis.

Signs, symptoms, and treatment of deficiency state

Signs and symptoms of hypocalcemia include paresthesias (pins and needles), increased neuromuscular excitability, muscle cramps, tetany, and convulsions. Bone fractures, bone

Calcium (continued)

pain, and loss of height may occur. These signs and symptoms are not specific to a calcium deficiency but may also be the result of a vitamin D deficiency (osteomalacia). Prolonged bed rest or immobilization can cause osteoporosis (loss of bone mass) because of loss of calcium from bones and increased urinary calcium excretion.

Use and effects of large doses

Calcium preparations are used in the treatment of hypocalcemia states (reduced ionized fraction). Oral ingestion of large quantities of a calcium salt is unlikely by itself to cause hypercalcemia. It has been suggested that high intake of calcium may prevent osteoporosis, although the results at present are equivocal (see Chapter 2).

Iodine

Physiology and biochemical pathways

Iodine is a trace element that is an integral part of the thyroid hormones thyroxine (T_4) and triiodothyronine (T_3). Thyroid hormones exert most if not all of their effects through the control of protein synthesis. Thyroid hormones have a calorigenic effect, a cardiovascular effect, metabolic effects, and an inhibitory effect on the secretion of thyrotropin by the pituitary.

Absorption

Iodine is readily absorbed from the diet and reaches circulation in the form of iodide. In circulation it is normally present in several forms, with 95% as organic iodine and approximately 5% as iodide. Most of the organic iodine is in thyroid hormone. Most T_4 and T_3 are transported in the plasma bound to carrier proteins. Only about 0.03% of the total thyroxine in plasma is free. Thyroxine-binding globulin is the major carrier of thyroid hormones. Some is also bound to thyroxine-binding prealbumin.

Metabolism and excretion

Iodine is metabolized in the thyroid gland by a series of steps beginning with uptake of iodide ion and ending with the release of T_4 and T_3 into the blood. T_4 is converted to T_3 in peripheral tissues. The liver is the major site of degradation of thyroid hormones. In humans, approximately 20% to 40% is eliminated in the feces. Thyroxine is eliminated slowly from the body with a half-life of 6 to 7 days. The intake and excretion of iodine are maintained in close balance.

Recommended dietary allowance and nutrient interactions

The daily iodine requirement for adults is about 1 to 2 µg/kg of body weight. The RDA for iodine is given in Table 1-1. Natural goitrogens present in certain foods (for example, cabbage, cassava, and mustard) may cause goiter in some areas.

Food sources

Seafoods and seaweeds are excellent sources of iodine. Most vegetable products are low in iodine. Dairy products and eggs have a variable content of iodine that depends upon the composition of the animal feed. Depending upon the process used, bread may be a source of iodine. The use of iodized salt in the United States provides a substantial source of iodine. Current levels of enrichment provide 76 µg of iodine per gram of salt. Approximately 10 to 12 g of iodized salt (or 3 to 5 g of sodium) are consumed in the United States per person per day.

Evaluation of nutritional status

The average urinary excretion of iodine in healthy adults is about 150 µg per day. Serum protein–bound iodine levels range from 4 to 8 µg/dl. Various thyroid function tests can reveal disorders of the thyroid.

Signs, symptoms, and treatment of deficiency

Iodine deficiency is a common worldwide cause of endemic goiter and cretinism in children. In the latter, the child is dwarfed, mentally retarded, and inactive, with a pug and expressionless face and an enlarged tongue. Successful treatment requires diagnosis long before these obvious signs appear. In the adult, reduced availability of iodine for thyroid hormone synthesis results in a compensatory enlargement of the thyroid gland (goiter). It is uncommon to see goiter due to iodine deficiency in the United States because of the use of iodized salt.

Treatment

Various thyroid hormone preparations are available to treat hypothyroidism and simple goiter.

Iodine (continued)

Use and effects of large doses

High intake of iodine may induce goiter because organification of iodine is blocked when the plasma iodine concentration exceeds 15 to 25 μg/ml. This has been documented in the Japanese, who have a high intake of seaweed. An intake in adults between 50 and 1000 μg/day of iodine is considered safe.

Iron

Physiology and biochemical pathways

With its presence in all cells, iron participates in a number of key biochemical reactions. It is present in compounds responsible for the transport of oxygen (hemoglobin and myoglobin), enzymes responsible for electron transport (cytochromes), and for the activation of oxygen (oxidases and oxygenases). A 70-kg adult man has about 2500 mg of iron in circulating hemoglobin and 500 to 1000 mg of iron in storage as ferritin or hemosiderin, largely in the liver, spleen, and bone marrow. The adult woman has about 1500 mg of iron in circulation and much lower stored iron, seldom exceeding 500 mg.

Absorption

The absorptive process is not fully understood. Iron is absorbed predominantly in the duodenum and lesser amounts in the remaining portion of the upper small intestine. Inorganic (nonheme) iron is absorbed with a low efficiency (<10%). Heme iron (from dietary hemoglobin and myoglobin) is more readily absorbed (10% to 20%). In general, healthy individuals absorb about 10% of dietary iron; iron-deficient individuals absorb between 10% and 20%. Ascorbic acid and meat in the diet will facilitate the absorption of nonheme iron. (Normal absorption is about 1 mg/day in men and 1.5 mg per day in women). Increased uptake occurs when there is iron deficiency, when iron stores are depleted, or when erythropoiesis is increased. Certain plant constituents such as oxalate, phytate, fiber, and tannin may reduce the absorption of nonheme iron. Reducing sugars, ascorbic acid, and heme increase the absorption of nonheme iron. Subjects with gluten-induced enteropathy or with achlorhydria absorb nonheme iron less efficiently from the diet. Antacids taken with meals also may reduce iron absorption.

Metabolism and excretion

Virtually all of the iron present in the erythrocytes is conserved and reutilized in the formation of new cells. Iron is transported in the plasma by transferrin and stored as ferritin or hemosiderin. This large protein may contain over 30% of its weight as iron. Hemosiderin represents aggregated ferritin molecules. Aside from menstrual losses in women, the daily loss of iron from skin, hair, sweat, intestinal desquamation, and urine amounts to about 0.9 mg/day in the adult. Menstrual losses average about 60 ml of blood per month, representing an additional loss of 0.5 mg/day of iron.

Recommended dietary allowance and nutrient interactions

Iron requirements are determined by obligatory physiological losses and the needs imposed by growth. Men have a requirement of about 1 mg of absorbed iron per day, whereas the menstruating woman requires about 1.5 mg/day. Postmenopausal women have a reduced need for iron, approximating that of men. Iron requirements are higher for the infant and during the last two trimesters of pregnancy. The infant frequently has inadequate intake because of the low iron content of milk and limited body stores of iron at birth. This is corrected by the introduction of iron-enriched cereals by 4 to 6 months of age. The RDA is shown in Table 1-1.

Food sources

Diets in the United States provide iron at about 6 mg/1000 kcal. Foods high in iron include organ meats such as liver and heart, wheat germ, egg yolks, oysters, fruits, and some dried beans. Lesser amounts are present in muscle meats, fish and fowl, and most green vegetables and cereals. Milk and milk products and most nongreen vegetables are low in iron. Heme iron contributes only 1 to 2 mg of iron per day in the average U.S. diet. Hence, nonheme iron is the main source of iron in the diet.

Iron (continued)

Evaluation of nutritional status

Hematocrit and hemoglobin determinations can establish the presence of anemia, but additional measurements are required to establish iron deficiency. For this purpose, measurements of serum ferritin levels are quite useful. Approximately 1 μg of ferritin per liter of serum is equivalent to 8 mg of stored iron. Hence, low serum ferritin levels are associated with depleted iron stores. However, infection, malignancy, and inflammatory disease may cause falsely high serum ferritin levels. A common laboratory finding suggestive of iron deficiency is a low serum iron level with an elevated total iron-binding capacity (TIBC), giving a low percentage of TIBC saturation. Peripheral blood smear morphology and bone marrow iron stains are also useful. Laboratory criteria for normal values of iron are shown in Table 2-9.

Signs, symptoms, and treatment of deficiency

Iron deficiency is one of the most common nutritional deficiencies in the world. Iron deficiency results in fatigue, pallor, tachycardia, listlessness, exertional dyspnea, burning sensation of the tongue, glossitis, and a hypochromic, microcytic anemia. Fatigue and impaired cognitive function and alertness may occur in early stages of iron deficiency, before anemia. Therapeutic supplementation with iron preparations is recommended when there is a clearly established iron deficiency. Orally administered ferrous sulfate is the preparation of choice in the treatment of iron deficiency. Administration for 6 months or longer is usually required to replenish bone marrow stores. Dietary changes should be made to include more iron-rich foods as well as ample intake of vitamin C to enhance iron absorption. Iron deficiency occurs most frequently in infancy and in menstruating and pregnant women. When iron deficiency occurs in men or in postmenopausal women, who have decreased iron requirements, bleeding should be investigated as a possible cause of the deficiency, because chronic blood loss will produce iron loss that will eventually lead to iron deficiency and anemia.

Use and effects of large doses

Excessive intake of medicinal or dietary iron may result in iron overload, a relatively rare condition called hemochromatosis. The normal person is able to control absorption of iron despite high intake. Only those with underlying disorders that augment iron absorption run the risk of hemochromatosis. However, large amounts of ferrous salts are toxic but rarely cause death in adults. Most deaths occur in the young, particularly those who are 12 to 24 months of age. For the young, as little as 1 to 2 g of iron may be fatal. Quick diagnosis and administration of deferoxamine have reduced the mortality rate from iron poisoning.

Magnesium

Physiology and biochemical pathways

The magnesium content in the adult human is about 24 g, with 60% found in the skeleton, 39% in the intracellular space (20% in skeletal muscle), and 1% in the extracellular space. Magnesium is associated with more than 300 different enzyme systems. Magnesium is essential to the metabolism of adenosine triphosphate (ATP) and as such participates in glucose utilization; synthesis of proteins, fats, and nucleic acids; muscle contraction; certain membrane transport systems; and nerve impulse transmission. Magnesium is highly concentrated in the mitochondria, where it is needed for oxidative phosphorylation. Red cells contain three times more magnesium than does serum.

Absorption

On the average, 35% to 45% of dietary magnesium is absorbed in the small intestine. Vitamin D and its metabolites have little or no effect on the intestinal absorption of magnesium. Absorption may be influenced by total magnesium intake; intestinal transit time; the amount of calcium, lactose and phosphate in the diet; and rate of water absorption. There is evidence to suggest that magnesium is absorbed by a carrier-mediated system and by simple diffusion, primarily at higher concentrations. Magnesium reenters the intestinal tract from bile and pancreatic and intestinal juices. Under normal conditions, nearly all is reabsorbed.

Metabolism and excretion

At least three different magnesium pools exist in the body, each with a different rate of turnover. The extracellular pool has a rapid turnover rate. The intracellular pool has a turnover rate about half that of the extracellular pool. The major pool, the skeleton, has a very slow turnover rate. In the plasma, 55% of the magnesium is in the free form, 13% in a complex form, and 32% in protein-bound forms. Approximately 60% to 70% of ingested magnesium is excreted in the feces, with most of the remainder excreted in the urine. An average of 1.4 mg of magnesium per kilogram of body weight is excreted daily in the urine.

Recommended dietary allowance and nutrient interactions

Magnesium and thiamin appear to interact. For example, thiamin administered to magnesium-deficient rats is not utilized and thiamin deficiency may develop. Calcium homeostasis is dependent upon magnesium in that severe hypomagnesemia prevents the release of parathyroid hormone and can cause hypocalcemia. The RDA for magnesium is 350 mg/day for men and 280 mg/day for women. During pregnancy and lactation, an extra allowance of 150 mg/day is recommended (see Table 1-1). Oriental diets and diets of vegetarians are high in magnesium.

Food sources

In the United States the average adult consumes 180 to 480 mg of magnesium daily. Grains and nuts are rich sources of magnesium. Meats, seafoods, and vegetables, especially green leafy types, are also good sources of magnesium. Magnesium present in the chlorophyll of plants appears readily available. Human milk contains 40 mg of magnesium per liter; cow's milk contains approximately 120 mg/L.

Evaluation of nutritional status

In magnesium deficiency, serum magnesium levels are markedly reduced, and urinary excretion is low. Atomic absorption spectroscopy is the easiest method to measure magnesium levels in urine or serum specimens.

Normal adult serum levels range from 1.6 to 2.6 mg/dl (0.65 to 1.05 mmol/L; 1.3 to 2.1 mEq/L). Urinary excretion levels for magnesium in the adult range from 36 to 207 mg/24 hours (1.5 to 9.5 mmol/24 hours; 3 to 17 mEq/L/24 hours).

Magnesium (continued)

Signs, symptoms, and treatment of deficiency

Magnesium deficiency may cause increased neuromuscular excitability, muscle spasms, and paresthesias. Prolonged deficiency can progress to tetany, seizures, and coma. Hypocalcemia and hypokalemia often accompany hypomagnesemia. Magnesium deficiency can be an associated complication of kwashiorkor. Hypomagnesemia is most often seen in alcoholics and in patients with fat malabsorption syndromes.

Use and effects of large doses

Magnesium sulfate (Epsom salt) at a dose of approximately 15 g is used for its laxative effect. Milk of magnesia and magnesium hydroxide and other magnesium salts are employed as gastric antacids. Because of the possibility of hypermagnesemia, their use should be avoided in individuals with impaired renal function.

Phosphorus

Physiology and biochemical pathways

The phosphorus content of an adult male is approximately 700 g, of which about 85% is found as bone minerals, calcium phosphate and hydroxyapatite. The remainder is in the cells and extracellular fluids as inorganic phosphate ions, phospholipids, phospho-proteins, and organic phosphoric esters. Most phosphorus is present as phosphate; no elemental phosphorus as such is present in the body. Phosphate is a constituent of nucleic acids and cell membranes and is an essential factor in all energy-producing reactions in the cells; it plays an important role in modifying concentrations of calcium in tissues, maintenance of acid-base equilibrium, and renal excretion of hydrogen ions.

Absorption

Phosphate is absorbed only from the small intestine by an active sodium-requiring transport process and to the largest extent by passive diffusion. Vitamin D stimulates phosphate absorption through a mechanism that is apparently separate from its action on calcium transport. Hence, in vitamin D deficiency, with a reduction in the availability of $1,25(OH)_2D_3$, absorption of phosphorus as well as calcium is reduced. When fed human milk, infants absorb 85% to 90% of the phosphorus present. When infants are fed cow's milk, which is seven times higher in phosphorus than human milk, the intestinal absorption of phosphorus is reduced to 65% to 70%. In older children and adults, with an intake of 1000 to 1500 mg of phosphorus, the efficiency of absorption is approximately 50% to 60%. Ingestion of aluminum-containing antacids reduces its absorption. The phosphorus in phytic acid, as present in cereal brans and unleavened breads, is unavailable for absorption.

Metabolism and excretion

Phosphate is present in plasma and extracellular fluids, in cell membranes, and in intra-cellular fluids. Serum concentrations of phosphate are higher in children than in adults. The higher serum concentration of phosphate during the growth period is important for mineralization of growing bone and cartilage. Phosphate absorbed from the intestine is readily excreted in the urine under the influence of parathyroid hormone, to maintain body phosphate balance. The majority of the phosphate in the plasma is in the ionic form (80%).

Recommended dietary allowance and nutrient interactions

The recommended dietary allowance for phosphorus, in milligrams per day, is the same as for calcium (with infants being an exception) and thereby provides a Ca:P ratio of 1.0. For the infant, evidence supports the recommendation of a dietary Ca:P ratio of about 1.5. A phosphorus intake greatly in excess of calcium, especially in the presence of a minimal intake of calcium, can reduce the availability of calcium and contribute to calcium deficiency. The recommended allowance for phosphorus is shown in Table 1-1.

Food sources

Phosphorus is abundant in the food supply. Most seafoods, nuts, grains, legumes, and cheeses are good sources (100 to 1200 mg/100 g of food item). Most green leafy vegetables, cauliflower, brussels sprouts, okra, potatoes, yams, and milk provide low amounts of phosphorus (50 to 100 mg per 100 g of food item).

Evaluation of nutritional status

Essentially, procedures to evaluate phosphorus status have been limited to measuring serum phosphorus levels. From a nutritional standpoint, interpretation of serum phos-phorus levels is difficult because of the numerous factors that may influence the serum level. In hospitalized patients, reduced serum levels occur most often because of rapid intravenous infusions of glucose. In outpatients, hypophosphatemia usually results from

Phosphorus (continued)

chronic use of aluminum-containing antacids. Other causes include rickets, hyperpara-thyroidism, sprue, and insulin therapy. Hypophosphatemia requires prompt diagnosis and treatment. Elevated serum phosphorus values have been observed to occur with hypo-parathyroidism, renal disease, diabetes, and healing fractures. The average serum phosphate of the normal adult is 3.5 mg/dl (2.5 to 4.0 mg/dl). Higher serum phosphate levels are observed in premature infants (7.9 mg/dl) and full-term infants (6.1 mg/dl), whereas values for children 1 to 10 years of age are lower (4.6 mg/dl).

Signs, symptoms, and treatment of deficiency

Phosphorus is abundant in a wide variety of foods. Consequently, nutritional deficiencies are rare. However, renal hypophosphatemia may occur in people with abnormalities of renal tubular function, thereby reducing tubular reabsorption of phosphate. Fanconi's syndrome may include hypophosphatemia. The major manifestations of chronic primary hypophosphatemia are growth retardation, skeletal deformities, and bone pain resulting from defective mineralization of bones. Phosphate depletion results in diminished concentration of intracellular organic phosphoric acid esters, including ATP and 2,3-diphosphoglycerate in red blood cells and ATP in muscle. Hemoglobin interacts with 2,3-diphosphoglycerate to promote oxygen release from oxyhemoglobin. Phosphate depletion may increase the rate of hemolysis of red blood cells, produce severe muscle weakness and ophthalmoplegia (see Figure 6-11), and diminish the phagocytic function of granulocytes.

Hypophosphatemia is particularly likely to occur in starved patients following re-feeding, in diabetic ketoacidosis patients following treatment with insulin and glucose, and in patients receiving high concentrations of glucose intravenously.

Use and effects of large doses

Phosphates are of limited therapeutic usefulness, although they may have a role in the management of the phosphate-depletion syndromes. Sodium phosphate has been employed to diminish hypercalcemia. Excess phosphate salts have a cathartic effect. Phosphate preparations are also used as urine acidifiers and antacids.

Zinc

Physiology and biochemical pathways

Zinc is essential for the function of more than 70 enzymes and is particularly essential for rapidly growing tissues. Deficiency will retard the synthesis of DNA, RNA, and protein, resulting in impaired cellular division, growth, and repair. DNA polymerase and RNA polymerase require zinc. Zinc is essential for sexual maturation, fertility and reproduction, night vision, sense of taste, and immune functions.

Absorption

Zinc is absorbed by an active process in the duodenum, jejunum, and probably to a lesser extent, in the ileum. Phytate and dietary fiber can reduce zinc absorption. The efficiency of zinc absorption depends on the type of meal eaten and the individual's zinc status; absorption may range from 10% to 40%. Fat malabsorption can reduce zinc absorption, and small-bowel diarrhea can result in losses of 12 to 17 mg of zinc per liter of diarrheal fluid.

Metabolism and excretion

After absorption, zinc is circulated bound to albumin (65%) and an α-macroglobulin (30%). Zinc is initially concentrated in the liver and then distributed to tissues. Zinc in the skeleton is relatively unavailable to other tissues.

The turnover of zinc in the body is slow, with a biological half-life of 250 days. The major route of excretion is in pancreatic and intestinal secretions, with only about 5% excreted daily in the urine. Depending on the ambient temperature or the presence of fever, up to 1 mg of zinc can be lost per liter of sweat.

Recommended dietary allowance and nutrient interactions

Excess zinc in the diet may decrease the absorption of copper. Recommended dietary intakes are given in Table 1-1.

Food sources

Meat, liver, eggs, and seafoods, especially oysters, are good sources of zinc. Whole-grain products (whole wheat or rye bread, oatmeal, whole corn) contain zinc, but it is less bioavailable in these food sources.

Evaluation of nutritional status

The laboratory criteria for evaluating zinc status are not well established. Various laboratory procedures include dark adaptation, taste acuity testing, and activities of zinc metalloenzymes such as alkaline phosphatase and carbonic anhydrase. Normal ranges of values for some of the laboratory measurements for zinc are shown below:

Zinc content of	Normal ranges
Serum	80-140 µg/dl
Red cell	40-44 µg/g hemoglobin
White cell	80-130 µg/10^{10} cells
Saliva (parotid)	23-70 ng/g
Sweat	0.55-1.75 mg/L
Nail	100-400 µg/g
Hair	100-230 µg/g
Urine	230-600 µg/day

Signs, symptoms, and treatment of deficiency

Clinical manifestations of zinc deficiency include growth retardation and hypogonadism, impaired taste and/or smell acuity, and poor wound healing. Mental lethargy, poor appetite, and dry, scaly skin may occur (Fig. 7-1). A reduction in immune competence is frequently noted. Nondietary zinc deficiency may be seen in cases of acrodermatitis

Zinc (continued)

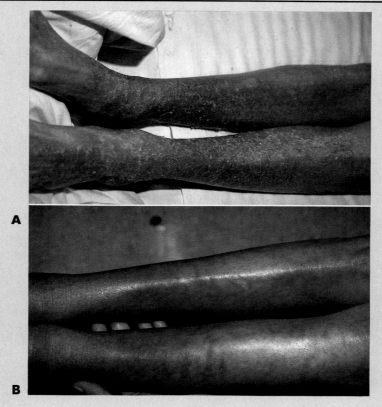

Fig. 7-1   Widespread scaling of the skin before **(A)** and after **(B)** treatment with zinc in a patient with fat malabsorption.

enteropathica, a rare inherited disorder that is responsive to zinc therapy, and with certain malabsorption syndromes.

Use and effects of large doses

Toxic effects of high doses of zinc are uncommon, although zinc may antagonize the metabolism of copper, and sickle cell anemia patients given approximately 150 mg of zinc daily may develop signs of copper deficiency. Plasma high-density lipoprotein cholesterol levels fall after the administration of high doses of zinc, and this may not be desirable.

The use of oral contraceptives may alter the postabsorptive utilization of zinc. However, evidence indicates that the requirement for zinc is not increased in women using these agents.

Other trace elements

Copper

Copper deficiency in the human is considered rare but is associated with Menke's disease, a genetic disorder in which copper utilization is impaired. Copper deficiency has been observed in infants fed only cow's milk. The clinical manifestations of copper deficiency include neutropenia, hypochromic microcytic anemia, depigmentation of skin and hair, neurological disturbances, lethargy, and abnormalities of connective tissue accompanied by skeletal abnormalities. The anemia resulting from copper deficiency is indistinguishable from iron-deficiency anemia. In the genetic Wilson's disease, copper accumulates in the liver, kidney, and brain, producing copper toxicity. Copper is a component of a number of metalloenzymes, including ceruloplasmin, lysyloxidase, cytochrome C, and superoxide dismutase. Copper plays a key role in iron absorption and mobilization. About 30% to 40% of the copper in the diet is absorbed. Liver, nuts, legumes, and oysters are good sources of copper. The copper requirement for adults is not well defined. A daily intake of 1.5 to 3 mg of copper by adults is considered safe and adequate. Normal serum levels of copper range from 90 to 125 μg/dl.

Chromium

Chromium is required for maintaining normal glucose metabolism, probably as a cofactor for insulin. Approximately 0.5% to 2% of inorganic chromium present in the diet is absorbed. Excretion is primarily in the urine. Glucose intolerance can result from chromium deficiency, such as patients on total parenteral nutrition without adequate chromium supplementation. The recommended allowance for chromium is 50 to 200 μg per day. There is no satisfactory test for the diagnosis of a chromium deficiency; diagnosis is based largely on documented clinical response to chromium—that is, improved glucose tolerance. For treatment, 200 μg/day of chromium as $CrCl_3$ orally or 10 g/day of brewer's yeast may be used. Meat products, eggs, cheese, whole grains, nuts, and brewer's yeast are good sources of chromium.

Manganese

The adult human body contains about 10 to 20 mg of manganese. Manganese-containing metalloenzymes are located primarily in mitochondria. Pyruvate carboxylase and manganese superoxide dismutase are examples of such enzymes. Manganese also functions as an enzyme cofactor and in the activation of glycosyl transferases, gluconeogenesis, lipid metabolism, and mucopolysaccharide metabolism. It may play a role in brain function through biogenic amine metabolism. Three to twelve percent of manganese is absorbed from the diet through the small intestine. Little is known of the clinical signs of deficiency, although a human man was reported to develop weight loss, hypocholesterolemia, dermatitis, nausea and vomiting, reddening of black hair, and reduced growth rate of hair when manganese was inadvertently omitted from a purified experimental diet. Sources of dietary manganese are mainly plant foods, with tea exceptionally high in the element. The RDA is listed in Table 1-2. Manganese toxicity has been reported in humans due to inhalation of dust or fumes from mining or various industrial operations.

Molybdenum

Molybdenum is an essential element for animals, although the effects of molybdenum on human health are not known with certainty. Molybdenum deficiency in humans is unknown. Molybdenum is a component of the metalloenzymes aldehyde oxidase, sulfite oxidase, and xanthine oxidase. Molybdenum in foods is readily absorbed, and more than half is excreted in the urine. Diets in the United States have been reported to provide 0.05 to 0.46 mg per day. Higher intakes of molybdenum may interfere with copper metabolism.

Other trace elements (continued)

Selenium

Selenium is a component of glutathione peroxidase, which protects cells and membranes against damage from peroxides when lipids are oxidized. Selenium in food is present largely in the form of amino acids, for example, selenomethionine. Selenium in food is readily absorbed. It is eliminated from the body largely by the kidney, although significant losses occur through the feces, breath, and skin. Low intakes of selenium result in lowered blood levels of selenium and may correlate with glutathione peroxidase activity in whole blood. Marginal intake occurs in the population of New Zealand and portions of the populations of China, Finland, and Venezuela. Individuals in areas of China where there is a low intake of selenium may develop a cardiomyopathy known as Keshan's disease, a disease that can be prevented with selenium supplementation. Various procedures have been employed to evaluate selenium status, including measuring urinary selenium levels, whole blood, erythrocyte and plasma selenium levels, and glutathione peroxidase activities of platelets or erythrocytes. No method is entirely satisfactory for assessing selenium status; thus, several techniques are usually employed. The RDA for selenium is 70 μg/day for men and 25 μg/day for women.

Fluorine

The importance of fluorine (known also as fluoride, the ionic form) is demonstrated in its ability to reduce dental caries and its influence on a number of biological processes. Fluoride is a normal component of calcified tissues. The fluoride ion is incorporated into the crystalline structure of hydroxyapatite of teeth to provide increased resistance to dental caries It is estimated that 50% to 80% of the fluoride in the human diet is absorbed.

An efficient renal excretion mechanism maintains blood fluoride concentrations within a narrow range, regardless of intake. The protective effects of fluoride against caries require a total dietary fluoride intake of 1.5 mg per day or more. A range between 1.5 and 2.5 mg in adolescents and between 1.5 and 4 mg in adults has been proved safe and adequate. Higher intake may result in mottling of the teeth. The Food and Nutrition Board of the National Academy of Sciences recommends fluoridation of public water supplies at 1 ppm if natural fluoride levels are low (see Chapter 2).

8

Case Studies

Alcohol Abuse and Nutrient Deficiencies

After loss of his job as a house painter, a 33-year-old man became severely depressed and spent most of his time alone. His already excessive intake of alcohol increased to the point that he was repeatedly in drunken stupors. Because of recurrent indigestion, he began taking aluminum-containing antacids throughout the day. Food intake was limited to canned soups, sodas, coffee, and four glasses or more of whole milk a day (to help relieve the indigestion). His weight remained relatively stable.

After 3 months, he was taken to the hospital by a friend who noted that he was disoriented to time and place and speaking "out of his head."

Physical examination: Weight for height was 90% of standard. Examination of his skin revealed no abnormalities. His tongue was slick (absence of papillae (see Fig. 6-7A). He had marked generalized weakness with foot drop (inability to raise his toes, see Fig. 6-10) and ataxia (difficulty balancing while standing or walking).

Laboratory data: Hematocrit 36%, mean cell volume 106 μ3 (normal 82 to 99), white blood cell count 4000/mm³ (normal 4000 to 11000/mm³) with several hypersegmented neutrophils noted on the peripheral blood smear.

TRUE or FALSE
1. The hypersegmented neutrophils support a diagnosis of vitamin C deficiency.
2. His riboflavin intake is probably well below the RDA.
3. The alcohol intake may have contributed to the development of his neuropathy by decreasing his absorption of thiamin.
4. He most likely will be found to have abnormal vitamin B_{12} absorption as the explanation for these hematologic abnormalities.
5. He almost definitely has thiamin deficiency.
6. He almost definitely has pellagra.
7. He almost definitely has iron deficiency.
8. He almost definitely has scurvy.
9. He almost definitely has zinc deficiency.

CASE
STUDY **4**   *Malabsorption Syndrome*

A 50-year-old woman underwent surgical resection of most of her small intestine after a vascular occlusion. Over the ensuing months, she lost a significant amount of weight despite a good appetite and a diet consisting of a variety of foods including fruits, vegetables, starches, meats, and fats. She had six to seven bowel movements per day, which she described as large, frothy, malodorous, and difficult to flush. She took no vitamin or mineral supplements but had been on oral antibiotics for treatment of a chronic sinus infection.

She had concerns about the weight loss and recurrences of bleeding into the skin (even without evident trauma) (Fig. 8-1) but otherwise felt well and had no complaints. Specifically, she denied muscle spasms, paresthesia (numbness and tingling), bone pain, and symptoms suggestive of night blindness.

Under these circumstances and on the basis of this information, which of the following statements is or are true?

1. A serum carotene level of 39 mg/dl (normal 50 to 300), if found, would indicate that she could not have been eating green and yellow-orange vegetables and fruits.
2. Vitamin C deficiency can be assumed to exist.
3. Bleeding into the skin may well reflect vitamin K deficiency in this case.
4. Her illness will increase her risk of developing zinc deficiency.
5. She is at increased risk for oxalate-containing kidney stones.
6. If her terminal (distal) ileum was in fact removed, she should be given a small daily supplement of vitamin B_{12} orally to prevent deficiency.

See Appendix A for answers and discussion.

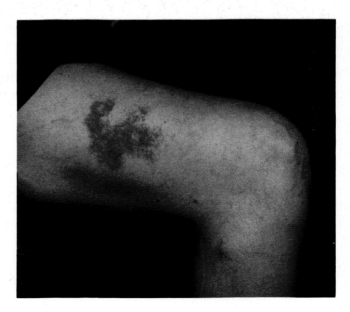

Fig. 8-1   Echymosis in a patient with fat malabsorption syndrome.

NUTRITION AND THE
HOSPITALIZED PATIENT

9

Nutrition and the Hospitalized Patient

PREVALENCE AND TYPES OF MALNUTRITION

Malnutrition can be either primary or secondary. *Primary malnutrition* is attributable only to altered or limited intakes of nutrients and is not associated with other disease states. *Secondary malnutrition* is defined as altered nutritional status as a result of an underlying disease process. Although primary malnutrition exists in certain areas of the United States and throughout the world, this section will emphasize secondary malnutrition in the hospitalized patient.

The era of nutrition support actually is quite young. In 1974 Butterworth wrote "The Skeleton in the Hospital Closet," focusing on iatrogenic (physician-induced) malnutrition in America. Other studies since 1974 have concluded that protein-calorie malnutrition affected approximately 44% of patients on a general medicine ward and 50% of general surgical patients. An additional study in 1979 of 134 consecutive admissions to a general medical ward revealed deterioration in nutritional status in 69% of the patients who remained hospitalized for 2 weeks or longer. Folate level, triceps skinfold, weight, arm muscle circumference, lymphocyte count, and hematocrit deteriorated in over 75% of patients who had normal admission values and who remained in the hospital for at least 2 weeks. Many nutritional parameters were abnormal at the time of discharge or transfer. In addition, patients with evidence of poor nutritional status had a significantly longer hospital stay and a higher mortality rate. The latter observations were reconfirmed in 1990.

In other studies, patients with reduced circulating protein levels were found to have a greater frequency of surgical complications. Patients with gastrointestinal carcinomas were randomized into a group fed with peripheral alimentation for 10 days prior to surgery and a control group who consumed a hospital diet. Both groups received postoperative parenteral nutrition. Mortality and major complications (including intraabdominal abscesses, peritonitis, anastomotic leaks, and paralytic ileus) were significantly lower in the group who received preoperative parenteral feedings. In addition, malnutrition has been linked to reduced lymphocyte counts and with anergy to skin tests. These abnormalities reflect increased susceptibility to infection and are reversible with nutritional repletion.

Findings such as these clearly indicate that indices of nutritional status have predictive value for a patient's hospital course and that nutritional repletion has benefits.

Table 9-1 Comparison of Marasmus and Kwashiorkor

Disease	Clinical setting	Time course to develop	Clinical features	Laboratory findings	Clinical course	Mortality
Marasmus	↓ Calorie intake	Months or years	Starved appearance Weight <80% standard for height Triceps skinfold <3 mm Midarm muscle circumference <15 cm	Creatinine-height index <60% standard	Reasonably preserved responsiveness to short-term stress	Low, unless related to underlying disease
Kwashiorkor	↓ Protein intake during stress state	Weeks	Well-nourished appearance Easy hair pluckability Edema	Serum albumin <2.8 g/dl Total iron-binding capacity <200 µg/dl Lymphocytes <1500/mm^3 Anergy	Infections Poor wound healing, decubitus ulcers, skin breakdown	High

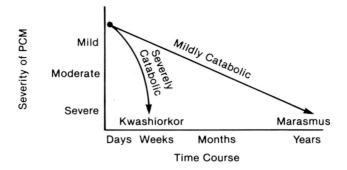

Fig. 9-1   Time course of protein-calorie malnutrition.

Common types of malnutrition in the hospital

Malnutrition in U.S. hospitals is usually attributable to an underlying disease process. However, actual development of malnutrition almost invariably is a result of failure to recognize and meet the increased nutritional needs of ill patients. By far the most common forms of malnutrition that are seen in the hospital are a result of protein deficiency, calorie deficiency, or both. Protein-calorie malnutrition appears in one or a combination of two types:
- Severe calorie deficiency, otherwise known as *marasmus*.
- A maladaptive state as a result of protein deficiency and stress, known as *kwashiorkor*.

The criteria for diagnosis of marasmus and kwashiorkor are found in Table 9-1, and their time course of development is shown in Figure 9-1.

Marasmus or severe cachexia

The diagnosis of marasmus is based on the physical finding of severe fat and muscle loss in the setting of prolonged caloric deficiency. Diminished skinfold thickness reflects the loss of calorie reserve (Figs. 9-2A–E); reduced arm muscle circumference with temporal and interosseous muscle wastage reflects the re-sorption of protein from the skeletal muscles and the heart. The laboratory picture is relatively unremarkable; occasionally the serum albumin level is reduced slightly, to about 2.8 g/dl. However, generally albumin levels are within the normal range. Despite a morose appearance, immunocompetence, wound heal-ing, and the ability to handle short-term stress are reasonably well preserved in most patients with marasmus.

Marasmus is a chronic rather than an acute illness, and it should be treated cautiously, the purpose being gradual reversal of the downward trend. Although nutritional support is necessary, overly aggressive repletion can result in severe, even life-threatening metabolic imbalances such as hypophosphatemia. When possible, the enteral route of nutritional support is preferred. Treatment should be started slowly to allow readaptation of metabolic and intestinal functions.

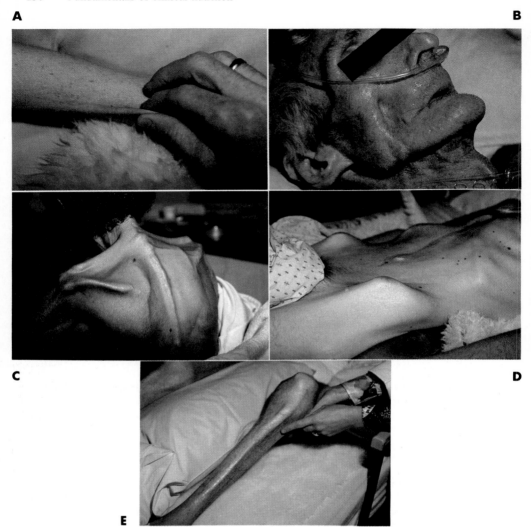

Fig. 9-2   (A–E) Losses of subcutaneous fat reserves and muscle mass in patients with marasmus.

Kwashiorkor

In contrast to marasmus, kwashiorkor is diagnosed largely on the basis of the laboratory results of tests on a patient in the acute state of poor protein intake and stress. In children, kwashiorkor is often the result of a starchy, low-protein diet while the child is under the stress of growth and parasitic or viral infection.

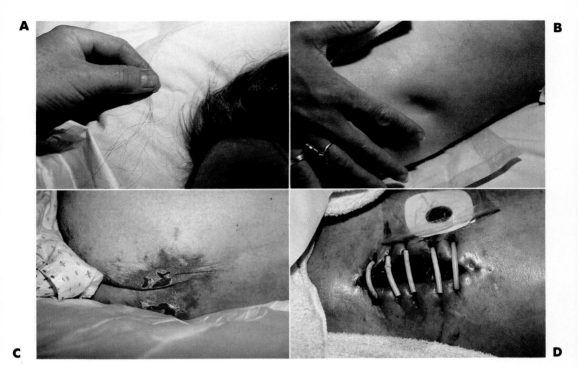

Fig. 9-3 (A–D) Clinical findings in kwashiorkor, including easy, painless hair pluckability, pitting edema, skin breakdown, and delayed wound healing.

In adults, kwashiorkor typically occurs in the hospitalized patient who is under acute stress and who is being supported with 5% dextrose solutions. Although the etiologic mechanisms are not understood, failure of the normal adaptive response of protein sparing that is seen in fasting may be an important factor. The time course of development may be as short as 2 weeks.

The clinical findings are often few. Fat reserves and muscle mass tend to be normal or even above normal, which gives the deceptive appearance of adequate nutrition. Signs that support the diagnosis of kwashiorkor include easily pluckable hair, transverse depigmentation of the hair, edema, skin breakdown and delayed wound healing (Figs. 9-3A–D). Characteristic laboratory changes include severely depressed levels of serum proteins such as albumin (<2.8 g/dl) and transferrin (<150 mg/dl) or reduced iron-binding capacity (<200 μg/dl). Associated with the fall in levels of circulating proteins is a depression of cellular immune function as reflected by lymphopenia (<1500 lymphocytes/mm^3 in adults and older children) and skin test anergy.

If full-blown kwashiorkor is diagnosed in the adult, the prognosis for recovery is poor, even with aggressive nutritional support. Dehiscence of surgical wounds is likely, host defenses are compromised, and death from overwhelming infection may occur despite antibiotic therapy. Unlike treatment for marasmus, parenteral feedings are often used in an attempt at rapid restoration of normal metabolic homeostasis. However, the metabolic state will not revert to completely normal until the underlying stress is removed. Although childhood kwashiorkor is often less foreboding, perhaps because of the lower degree of stress required to precipitate the deficiency state, in both the adult and the child the prognosis is poor. Kwashiorkor is prevented much more easily than it is treated. Prevention depends on early recognition of a severely stressed (hypermetabolic) state and then replacement of calculated calorie and protein needs.

Marasmic kwashiorkor

The combined form of protein-calorie malnutrition develops when the acute stress of surgery or trauma is experienced by the chronically starved patient. A life-threatening situation can occur because of the high risk of infection and other complications. If kwashiorkor predominates, the need for vigorous nutritional therapy is urgent. It is of utmost importance to determine the major component of protein-calorie malnutrition so the appropriate nutritional plan can be developed, because the starved, unstressed (hypometabolic) patient is at risk of complications of overfeeding, and the stressed patient at risk for kwashiorkor is more likely to suffer from underfeeding.

SELECTED READING

Prevalence and Types of Malnutrition

Bistrian BR, Blackburn GL, Hallowell EH, et al: Protein status of general surgical patients, *JAMA* 230(6):858-860, 1974.

Bistrian BR, Blackburn GJ, Vitale J, et al: Prevalence of malnutrition in general medical patients *JAMA* 235(15):1567-1570, 1976.

Butterworth CE: The skeleton in the hospital closet, *Nutr Today* 9:4-8, 1974.

Weinsier RL, Hunker EM, Krumdieck CL, et al: Hospital malnutrition: a prospective evaluation of general medical patients during the course of hospitalization, *Am J Clin Nutr* 32(2):418-428, 1979.

10

Nutritional Assessment

Many physical and laboratory findings are a reflection of underlying disease as well as nutritional status. Therefore, the evaluation of a patient's nutritional status depends on an integration of several parts to form the whole. The complete nutrition evaluation includes the history, physical examination, anthropometrics, and laboratory evaluation.

Each medical and surgical subspecialty has certain historical questions and clinical and laboratory assessment parameters that are pertinent. Similarly, clinical nutrition has a specialized history review, physical examination, and laboratory approach, which are all critical to a complete nutritional assessment.

Nutritional history

The nutritional history is geared to identifying underlying mechanisms that put patients at risk for nutritional depletion or excess. These mechanisms include the following:
- Inadequate intake
- Inadequate absorption
- Decreased utilization
- Increased losses
- Increased requirements

This systematic approach to the nutritional history screen is outlined in Table 10-1.

People who are at particular risk for nutritional deficiencies from one of a variety of mechanisms include those who are
- Grossly underweight: weight for height below 80% of standard.
- Grossly overweight: weight for height above 120% of standard (Due to the tendency to overlook protein and calorie needs of the acutely ill obese patient).
- Experiencing recent loss of 10% or more of usual body weight.
- Alcoholic.
- Taking nothing by mouth for more than 10 days while being given simple intravenous solutions.
- Experiencing protracted nutrient losses: malabsorption syndromes, short-gut syndromes/fistulas, renal dialysis, draining abscesses, or wounds.
- Experiencing increased metabolic needs: extensive burns, infection, trauma, or protracted fever.
- Taking drugs with antinutrient or catabolic properties: steroids, immunosuppressants, or antitumor agents.

Table 10-1   Nutritional history screen—a systematic approach to the detection of deficiency syndromes

Mechanism of deficiency	If history of	Suspect deficiency of
Inadequate intake	Alcoholism	Calories, protein, thiamin, niacin, folate, pyridoxine, riboflavin
	Avoidance of fruit, vegetables, grains	Vitamin C, thiamin, niacin, folate
	Avoidance of meat, dairy products, eggs	Protein, vitamin B_{12}
	Constipation, hemorrhoids, diverticulosis	Dietary fiber
	Isolation, poverty, dental disease, food idiosyncrasies	Various nutrients
	Weight loss	Calories, other nutrients
Inadequate absorption	Drugs (especially antacids, anticonvulsants, cholestyramine, laxatives, neomycin, alcohol)	(See Appendix C "Drug/Nutrient interactions")
	Malabsorption (diarrhea, weight loss, steatorrhea)	Vitamins A, D, K, calories, protein, calcium, magnesium, zinc
	Parasites	Iron, vitamin B_{12} (fish tapeworm)
	Pernicious anemia	Vitamin B_{12}
	Surgery	
	Gastrectomy	Vitamin B_{12}, iron
	Resection of small intestine	Vitamin B_{12} (if distal ileum), others as in malabsorption
Decreased utilization	Drugs (especially anticonvulsants, antimetabolites, oral contraceptives, isoniazid, alcohol)	(See Appendix C "Drug/Nutrient Interactions")
	Inborn errors of metabolism (by family history)	Various nutrients
Increased losses	Alcohol abuse	Magnesium, zinc
	Blood loss	Iron
	Centesis (ascitic, pleural taps)	Protein
	Diabetes, uncontrolled	Calories
	Diarrhea	Protein, zinc, electrolytes
	Draining abscesses, wounds	Protein, zinc
	Nephrotic syndrome	Protein, zinc
	Peritoneal dialysis or hemodialysis	Protein, water-soluble vitamins, zinc

Table 10-1   Nutritional history screen—a systematic approach to the detection of deficiency syndromes (continued)

Mechanism of deficiency	If history of	Suspect deficiency of
Increased requirements	Fever	Calories
	Hyperthyroidism	Calories
	Physiologic demands (infancy, adolescence, pregnancy, lactation)	Various nutrients
	Surgery, trauma, burns, infection	Calories, protein, vitamin C, zinc
	Tissue hypoxia	Calories (inefficient utilization)
	Cigarette smoking	Vitamin C, folic acid

The presence of any one characteristic is a warning that a patient is at increased risk for malnutrition, but the absence of these characteristics does not mean that malnutrition does not exist or cannot occur.

Physical examination

Physical findings that suggest vitamin, mineral, and protein-calorie deficiencies and excesses are outlined in Table 10-2. A common theme running through the nutrition physical examination is that rapidly proliferating tissues are likely to show signs of nutrient deficiency or excess. Therefore, hair, skin, and tongue papillae are particularly likely to reveal nutritional problems. Most of the physical findings are not specific for an individual nutrient deficiency. Therefore, the history, physical examination, and anthropometric data must be integrated to make a diagnosis.

Anthropometrics

Anthropometrics describe body morphology by a series of measurements. Those most commonly used are body weight, height, triceps skinfold, and midarm muscle circumference (Figs. 10-1 and 10-2). Height is used to calculate energy needs in the Harris-Benedict equation and for measures such as the creatinine-height index.

Evaluation of normal body weight is often based on the Metropolitan Height-Weight Charts shown in Chapter 2, Table 2-1. The weight guidelines were published in both 1959 and 1983, with the 1983 weight standards being significantly higher than the 1959 standards. However, because of certain inappropriate assumptions that were made in preparation of the 1983 tables, the 1959 chart is still preferred. (See Chapter 2 for further discussion.)

When a patient is admitted to the hospital, or soon thereafter, weight and height are determined and plotted on a reference graph. A graph is routinely kept in pediatric wards to document growth rate, but it is equally important for

Table 10-2   Clinical nutrition examination

Clinical findings	Consider deficiency of*	Consider excess of	Frequency†
Hair, nails			
Flag sign (transverse depig-mentation of hair)	Protein		Rare
Easily pluckable hair	Protein		Common
Sparse hair	Protein, biotin, zinc	Vitamin A	Occasional
Corkscrew hairs and une-merged coiled hairs	Vitamin C		Common
Transverse ridging of nails	Protein		Occasional
Skin			
Scaling	Vitamin A, zinc, essential fatty acids	Vitamin A	Occasional
Cellophane appearance	Protein		Occasional
Cracking (flaky paint or crazy pavement dermatosis)	Protein		Rare
Follicular hyperkeratosis	Vitamins A, C		Occasional
Petechiae (especially perifol-licular)	Vitamin C		Occasional
Purpura	Vitamins C, K		Common
Pigmentation, desquamation of sun-exposed areas	Niacin		Rare
Yellow pigmentation–sparing sclerae (benign)		Carotene	Common
Eyes			
Papilledema		Vitamin A	Rare
Night blindness	Vitamin A		Rare
Perioral			
Angular stomatitis	Riboflavin, pyri-doxine, niacin		Occasional
Cheilosis (dry, cracking, ul-cerated lips)	Riboflavin, pyri-doxine, niacin		Rare
Oral			
Atrophic lingual papillae (slick tongue)	Riboflavin, nia-cin, folate, vitamin B_{12}, protein, iron		Common

*In this table, *protein deficiency* is used to signify kwashiorkor.
†These frequencies are an attempt to reflect the authors' experience in the setting of a U.S. medical practice. Findings common in other countries but virtually unseen in usual medical practice settings in the United States (e.g., xerophthalmia and endemic goiter) are not listed.

Table 10-2   Clinical nutrition examination (continued)

Clinical findings	Consider deficiency of*	Consider excess of	Frequency†
Glossitis (scarlet, raw tongue)	Riboflavin, niacin, pyridoxine, folate, vitamin B_{12}		Occasional
Hypogeusesthesia, hyposmia	Zinc		Occasional
Swollen, retracted, bleeding gums (if teeth are present)	Vitamin C		Occasional
Bones, joints			
Beading of ribs, epiphyseal swelling, bowlegs	Vitamin D		Rare
Tenderness (subperiosteal hemorrhage in child)	Vitamin C		Rare
Neurologic			
Headache		Vitamin A	Rare
Drowsiness, lethargy, vomiting		Vitamins A, D	Rare
Dementia	Niacin, vitamin B_{12}		Rare
Confabulation, disorientation	Thiamin (Korsakoff's psychosis)		Occasional
Ophthalmoplegia	Thiamin, phosphorus		Occasional
Peripheral neuropathy (e.g., weakness, paresthesias, ataxia, and decreased tendon reflexes, fine tactile sense, vibratory sense, and position sense)	Thiamin, pyridoxine, vitamin B_{12}	Pyridoxine	Occasional
Tetany	Calcium, magnesium		Occasional
Other			
Parotid enlargement	Protein (also consider bulimia)		Occasional
Heart failure	Thiamin (wet beriberi), phosphorus		Occasional
Sudden heart failure, death	Vitamin C		Rare
Hepatomegaly	Protein	Vitamin A	Rare
Edema	Protein, thiamin		Common
Poor wound healing, decubitus ulcers	Protein, vitamin C, zinc		Common

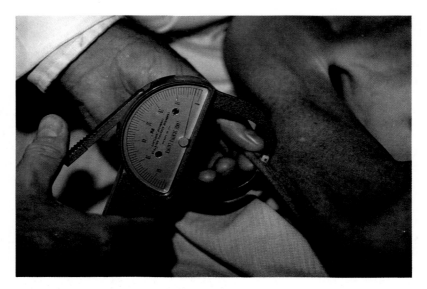

Fig. 10-1 Measurement of the triceps skinfold with Lange skinfold calipers.

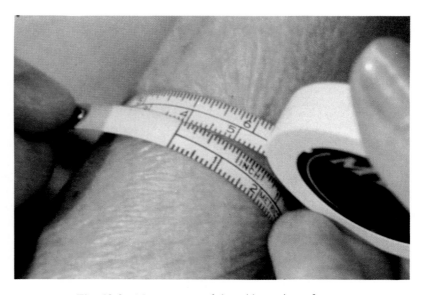

Fig. 10-2 Measurement of the midarm circumference.

adults because it allows documentation of nutritional risk on admission and any change in status that occurs during hospitalization. Adult patients who are 20% or more above standard weight are likely to be grossly overweight regardless of their body frame type. Those who are 20% or more below standard are likely to be grossly underweight and at high risk of nutritional deficiency.

Body weight is one of the most convenient and useful indicators of nutritional status. Weight loss that is not secondary to fluid loss is an ominous sign in the hospitalized patient. Such loss likely reflects the use of body protein (i.e., muscle and organ tissue) as a metabolic fuel, which occurs quickly when calorie intake is severely restricted. This occurs in patients who are maintained on intravenous solutions of 5% and 10% glucose. The obese patient can suffer extreme protein-calorie malnutrition under such circumstances while maintaining the appearance of being well fed. In general, the acutely ill obese patient should not be treated with caloric restriction. Conversely, weight maintenance may falsely reflect adequate nutritional support if fluid, as a result of edema (a common feature of protein-calorie malnutrition) replaces fat and muscle tissue.

There are numerous ways to determine body fat stores. Because approximately 50% of body fat stores are subcutaneous, one convenient method uses skinfold measurements. Although a variety of sites can be used, the triceps skinfold is a convenient site that is thought to be representative of the fatness of the entire body. The triceps skinfold measurement is taken at the midpoint of the upper arm using a set of skinfold calipers. Normal and abnormal triceps skinfold values are presented in Table 10-3A.

Assessment of skeletal muscle mass is frequently accomplished using the midarm muscle circumference (MAMC). A soft tape measure is used to determine the circumference of the mid upper arm. The MAMC is calculated with the following formula, where

AC = arm-muscle circumference in centimeters

and

TSF = triceps skinfold thickness in centimeters:
$$MAMC = AC - (3.14 \times TSF)$$

A guideline for interpreting the MAMC is shown in Table 10-3B.

Laboratory studies

Any of a large number of routine and specialized laboratory tests can yield useful information for evaluating nutritional status. Table 10-4 outlines relevant laboratory tests and their interpretation. It is important to note that many of the tests are not specific for nutritional status but do reflect the medical status of the patient also. The following are examples of tests that are of particular usefulness and have different nutritional significance.

Creatinine-height index. The creatinine-height index is a laboratory measurement used to estimate skeletal muscle mass. Creatine phosphate is a high-energy compound in the skeletal muscle that is nonenzymatically dephosphorylated to form creatinine. The amount of creatinine excreted in a 24-hour urine

Table 10-3A   Triceps skinfold thickness in adults

Percent of standard	Men (mm)	Women (mm)	Calorie reserves
100	12.5	16.5	
90	11.0	15.0	
80	10.0	13.0	Adequate
70	9.0	11.5	
60	7.5	10.0	
50	6.0	8.0	
40	5.0	6.5	Borderline
30	4.0	5.0	
20	2.5	3.0	Severely depleted

Table 10-3B   Midarm muscle circumference in adults

Percent of standard	Men (cm)	Women (cm)	Muscle mass
100	25.5	23.0	Adequate
90	23.0	21.0	
80	20.0	18.5	Borderline
70	18.0	16.0	
60	15.0	14.0	
50	12.5	11.5	Severely depleted
40	10.0	9.0	

sample depends on skeletal muscle mass (see Table 10-4). As an approximation, women excrete 18 mg/kg/day and men excrete 23/mg/kg/day.

The creatinine-height index represents a comparison between actual 24-hour creatinine excretion and standard 24-hour creatinine excretion for a given height. Table 10-5 shows predicted urinary creatinine values for adult men and women. Values of 80% to 100% indicate adequate muscle mass, values of 60% to 80% indicate a moderate deficit, whereas values of less than 60% indicate a severe deficit of muscle mass.

Visceral protein compartment. The visceral protein compartment is composed of proteins that act as carriers, binders, and immunologically active proteins. Several circulating proteins that are used to estimate the size of the visceral compartment include albumin, transferrin (or total iron-binding capacity), thyroxine-binding prealbumin, and retinol-binding protein. Because their half-lives differ considerably (e.g., half-life of albumin is about 21 days, whereas that of

Table 10-4   Laboratory tests and values*

SERUM ALBUMIN

Normal	3.5-5.5 g/dl
Nutritional use	2.8–3.5: Compromised protein status
	<2.8: Possible kwashiorkor
	Increasing value reflects positive nitrogen balance

Other causes of low value
  Common

Infection and other stress, especially with poor
    protein intake
Burns, trauma
Congestive heart failure
Fluid overload
Recumbency
Severe hepatic insufficiency

  Uncommon

Nephrotic syndrome
Zinc deficiency
Bacterial overgrowth of small bowel

Causes of normal value
  despite malnutrition

Dehydration
Infusion of albumin, fresh frozen plasma, whole
    blood

TOTAL IRON-BINDING CAPACITY

Normal	270-400/μg/dl
Nutritional use	<270: Compromised protein status
	<200: Possible kwashiorkor
	Increasing value reflects positive nitrogen balance
	More labile than albumin

Other causes of low value

Similar to albumin

Cause of normal or high
  value despite malnutri-
  tion

Iron deficiency

BLOOD UREA NITROGEN (BUN)

Normal	8-23 mg/dl
Nutritional use	Evaluation of protein intake; if serum creatinine is normal, use BUN; if serum creatinine is elevated, use BUN/creatinine

Ratio

<8: Poor protein intake
>12: Possibly adequate protein intake

Other causes of low value

Severe liver disease
Anabolic state

---

*Actual normal value ranges will vary depending upon laboratory standards.   *Continued.*

Table 10-4   Laboratory tests and values—cont'd

BLOOD UREA NITROGEN (BUN)–cont'd.

Causes of high value despite poor protein intake	Renal failure (use BUN/creatinine ratio) Congestive heart failure Gastrointestinal hemorrhage Corticosteroid therapy Dehydration Shock

SERUM CREATININE

Normal	0.6-1.6 mg/dl
Nutritional use	<0.6: Muscle wasting due to calorie deficiency
Causes of high value despite muscle wasting	Renal failure Severe dehydration

PROTHROMBIN TIME (PT)

Normal	<1-2 sec beyond control, or 70%-100% of control activity
Nutritional use	Prolongation: vitamin K deficiency
Other causes of prolonged value	Anticoagulant therapy: warfarin (Coumadin) Severe liver disease

TOTAL LYMPHOCYTE COUNT

Total lymphocyte count (TLC) = (white blood cell count) × (% lymphocytes)	
Normal	>1500/mm³
Nutritional use	<1500: possible immunocompromise associated with protein-calorie malnutrition, especially kwashiorkor
Significant limitation	Marked day-to-day fluctuation
Other causes of low TLC	Severe stress, e.g., infections, with left shift Corticosteroid therapy Renal failure Cancer, e.g., colon
Causes of high TLC despite malnutrition	Infections Leukemia, myeloma Cancer, e.g., stomach, breast Adrenal insufficiency

24-HOUR URINARY CREATININE

Normal	800-1800 mg/day; reflects muscle mass; standardized for height and sex

Table 10-4   Laboratory tests and values—cont'd

24-HOUR URINARY CREATININE–cont'd.

Nutritional use	Low value: muscle wasting due to calorie deficiency
Other causes of low value	Incomplete urine collection Increasing serum creatinine
Causes of normal or high value despite malnutrition	>24-hour collection Decreasing serum creatinine

24-HOUR URINARY UREA NITROGEN (UUN)

Normal	<5 g/day—depends on level of protein intake

Nutritional use	Determine level of catabolism
	Estimate nitrogen (protein) balance (EPB)
	   EPB = protein intake − protein loss
	   Protein loss = [24-hr UUN (g) + 4] × 6.25

Exception	Additional factors in burn patients and others with large nonurinary nitrogen losses
Causes of low UUN	Low protein intake Active fluid retention Increasing BUN Incomplete urine collection
Causes of high UUN	High protein intake Stress Corticosteroid therapy Active diuresis Decreasing BUN >24-hour urine collection

RED BLOOD CELL PARAMETERS

Normal	
Hemoglobin	Female: 12-15 g/dl Male: 14-17 g/dl
Hematocrit	Female: 34%-44% Male: 39%-49%
Mean corpuscular volume (MCV)	82-99 μ3
Nutritional use of hemoglobin and hematocrit	Low value indicates anemia, possibly due to nutritional deficiency
Nutritional use of MCV	
<82 (Microcytic)	Iron, copper, pyridoxine deficiency
82-99 (normocytic)	Kwashiorkor
≥100 (macrocytic)	Folate, vitamin B_{12} deficiency

Table 10-5   Predicted urinary creatinine values—adults

Men*		Women†	
Height	Predicted creatinine (mg/24 hr)	Height	Predicted creatinine (mg/24 hr)
5′ 2″ (157.5 cm)	1288	4′10″ (147.3 cm)	830
5′ 3″ (160.0)	1325	4′11″ (149.9)	851
5′ 4″ (162.6)	1359	5′ 0″ (152.4)	875
5′ 5″ (165.1)	1386	5′ 1″ (154.9)	900
5′ 6″ (167.6)	1426	5′ 2″ (157.5)	925
5′ 7″ (170.2 cm)	1467	5′ 3″ (160.0 cm)	949
5′ 8″ (172.7)	1513	5′ 4″ (162.6)	977
5′ 9″ (175.3)	1555	5′ 5″ (165.1)	1006
5′10″ (177.8)	1596	5′ 6″ (167.6)	1044
5′11″ (180.3)	1642	5′ 7″ (170.2)	1076
6′ 0″ (182.9 cm)	1691	5′ 8″ (172.7 cm)	1109
6′ 1″ (185.4)	1739	5′ 9″ (175.3)	1141
6′ 2″ (188.0)	1785	5′10″ (177.8)	1174
6′ 3″ (190.5)	1831	5′11″ (180.3)	1206
6′ 4″ (193.0)	1891	6′ 0″ (182.9)	1240

80% to 100% = acceptable; 60% to 80% = moderate depletion; <60% = severe depletion.
*Creatinine coefficient (men) = 23 mg/kg of ideal body weight/24 hours.
†Creatinine coefficient (women) = 18 mg/kg of ideal body weight/24 hours.
From Blackburn GL, et al: Nutritional and metabolic assessment of the hospitalized patient, *JPEN* 1:11, 1977.

Table 10-6   Classification of patients according to catabolic state by 24-hour urine urea nitrogen values*

Degree of catabolism	Clinical setting	Nitrogen loss
Normal		<5 g
Mild	Elective surgery	5-10 g
Moderate	Infection; major surgery	10-15 g
Severe	Severe sepsis; major burns	>15 g

*Because urea nitrogen excretion increases with increased protein intake, the values in this table apply only if intake is below the amount of the estimated protein loss by ≥10 g.

retinol-binding protein is closer to 12 hours), some will reflect changes in nutritional status more quickly than others. The serum albumin level is a convenient laboratory test and is most commonly used despite its long half-life. A drop in circulating levels of proteins such as albumin and transferrin often accompanies significant physiological stress, as from infection or injury, and is not necessarily an indication of malnutrition. On the other hand, adequate nutritional support of calorie and protein needs is critical for the return of these proteins to normal

Table 10-7   Reference values for vitamin levels

Carotene	79-233 µg/dl
Vitamin A	25-70 µg/dl
Thiamin	1-1.23 A/C*—acceptable
	>1.23 A/C—deficient
Riboflavin	1-1.67 A/C*—acceptable
	>1.67 A/C—deficient
Pyridoxine	1.15-1.89 A/C*—acceptable
	>1.89 A/C—deficient
Folic acid, serum	3-10 ng/ml
Folic acid, red cell	>160 ng/ml
Vitamin B$_{12}$	200-700 pg/ml
Vitamin C	0.5-1.5 mg/dl

*The activity coefficient (A/C) is a ratio of enzyme activity in a sample, with or without the addition of coenzyme to the system. Therefore, the higher the A/C, the lower the vitamin level, and the lower the A/C, the higher the vitamin level.
Source: Clinical Vitamin Laboratory, University of Alabama at Birmingham.

levels as the stress resolves. Thus, low values by themselves do not define malnutrition but often point toward an increased risk of malnutrition due to stress. Failure of levels to rise as stress resolves most likely indicates inadequate nutritional support.

Urinary urea nitrogen. The 24-hour urine collection for urea nitrogen content is used to assess the degree of protein catabolism and protein balance. The amount of protein catabolized in 24 hours is reflected by the amount of urea produced. Under normal circumstances, virtually all of this appears as urinary urea nitrogen (UUN). A small amount of protein is lost as nonurea nitrogen in the urine and in sweat, hair, skin, and stool. These additional daily losses are estimated using a fudge factor of 4 g of nitrogen. Total nitrogen losses are then converted to protein by multiplying by 6.25. Thus:

Protein loss = [24-hour UUN (g) + 4] × 6.25

The difference between intake and loss of protein is protein balance. When protein intake is small (<about 20 g/day), the above formula indicates the severity of the catabolic state (Table 10-6). With adequate intake of calories, protein losses can be matched and protein balance can be achieved.

Vitamin and mineral assays. The detection of a vitamin deficiency by laboratory tests is desirable because a vitamin deficiency may predate more serious clinical complications. Vitamin assays also confirm clinical impressions and indicate important drug-nutrient interactions. Vitamin assays and normal values are given in Table 10-7.

Tests of immune function. The body's defenses against infection are divided into three main categories: mechanical, cellular, and humoral. Mechanical defenses permit the body to protect itself from microbial invasion by intact epithelial surfaces, mucus barriers, and digestive enzymes. Epithelial cells, like all others, require an adequate supply of nutrients for growth, turnover, and function. Cellular defense mechanisms are mediated by lymphocytes and plasma cells and by polymorphonuclear leukocytes, which ingest and destroy bacteria or foreign bodies. Humoral defense mechanisms are mediated by gamma globulins or other plasma proteins that help to destroy microorganisms. Some antibodies appear in secretions such as tears, colostrum, and intestinal mucus.

There is ample evidence that all of these defense systems are impaired in protein-calorie malnutrition. Protein malnutrition is commonly associated with low reactivity to skin tests (such as mumps skin test), low visceral protein levels, and low lymphocyte counts. Furthermore, with nutritional repletion, immunocompetence can be restored.

SELECTED READING

Nutritional assessment

Grant JP, Custer PB, Thurlow J: Current techniques of nutritional assessment, *Surg Clin North Am* 61(3):437-463, 1981.
Hall CA: Nutritional assessment (letter), *N Engl J Med* 307:754-755, 1982.
McLaren DS: Clinical manifestations of nutritional disorders. In Shils ME, Young VR, editors: *Modern nutrition in health and disease,* ed 7, Philadelphia, 1988, Lea and Febiger, 733-745.
Weinsier RL, Heimburger DC, Butterworth CE Jr: *Handbook of clinical nutrition,* ed 2, St Louis, 1989, CV Mosby.

11

Nutritional Support

General guidelines for feeding the hospitalized patient
Therapeutic diets
Enteral feeding
Parenteral nutrition

GENERAL GUIDELINES FOR FEEDING THE HOSPITALIZED PATIENT

Decisions about nutritional repletion, or refeeding, involve the method of eating as well as the rapidity of refeeding and the goals for protein and calorie intake. The feeding quadrangle (Fig. 11-1) demonstrates that feeding can either be parenteral, which completely circumvents the gastrointestinal (GI) tract, or enteral. With one or a combination of approaches, virtually every patient can be supported nutritionally.

Calculating calorie needs and refeeding

Calorie needs are difficult to determine on an individual basis. Marked variations occur from person to person, and disease states can dramatically alter calorie requirements. An indirect calorimeter or a metabolic cart can be used to establish caloric needs.

The Harris-Benedict equation allows an estimation of the basal energy expenditure (BEE) using the formulas or nomogram given in Figures 11-2A and B. Actual calorie requirements are estimated by multiplying this BEE value by a factor that allows for activity and stress of illness. For most hospitalized patients, calorie needs will be reasonably approximated in the range of BEE × (1.2 to 1.5). The lower value is used for patients without evidence of

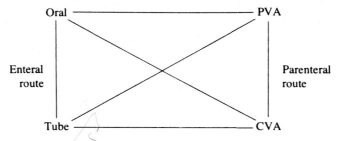

Fig. 11-1 The feeding quadrangle. PVA = peripheral venous alimentation; CVA = central venous alimentation.

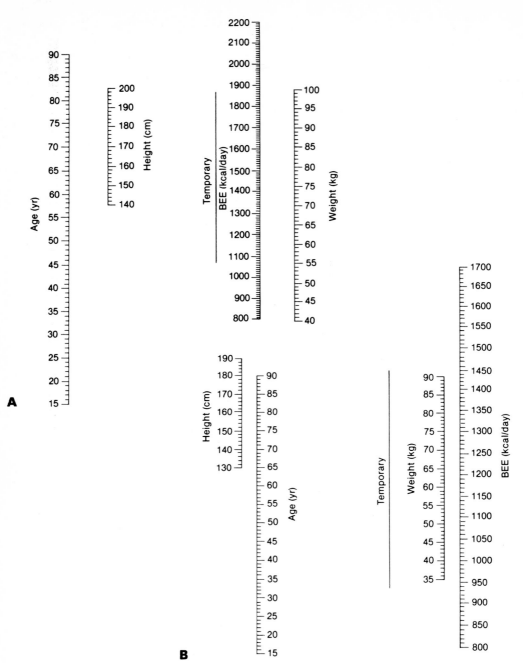

Fig. 11-2 A, Nomogram for calculating basal energy expenditure for men. **B,** Nomogram for calculating basal energy expenditure for women. Directions: 1. Locate the height and weight on the scale, placing a straight edge (ruler) between these points, intersecting the temporary variable line. 2. Holding a pencil at the point of intersection (on temporary variable line), locate the age, and pivot ruler to this point on the age scale. The point of intersection on the BEE scale is the predicted BEE. (From Rainey-MacDonald CG et al: The Harris-Benedict equations, *JPEN* 6:59, 1982.)

Table 11-1   Calorie goals in refeeding the hypometabolic-starved patient

Days	Calories related to basal energy expenditure (BEE)
1, 2	BEE × 0.8
3, 4	BEE × 1.0
4-6	BEE × 1.2 to 1.5
6 and after	BEE × 2.0 if weight gain is desired

Table 11-2   Selective approaches to nutritional support

Patient type	Aim	Nutritional support	Risks of overfeeding	Error likely
Hypometabolic, starved	Rebuild	Cautious, with portion of fuel as fat	Hypophosphatemia, repletion heart failure	Commission (overzealous support)
Hypermeta-bolic, stressed	Replace	Aggressive but not ex-cessive	↑ O$_2$ consumption and CO$_2$ produc-tion	Omission (in-adequate support)

significant physiologic stress; the upper value is used for patients with marked stress, such as from widespread infection or severe trauma. The aim in hypermetabolic patients is to *replace* calorie and protein needs.

In certain situations, values outside this range are recommended. Chronically starved patients without evidence of acute stress (i.e., hypometabolic) should be approached cautiously, with the aim of providing no more than their BEE the first day and gradually increasing to meet calorie needs in the course of about 5 days. (This is to avoid precipitating serious complications of refeeding such as hypophosphatemia or repletion heart failure.) After stabilization at this level, calorie intake can be increased up to BEE × 2.0 in order to achieve weight gain. Table 11-1 summarizes the refeeding of the hypometabolic patient. Table 11-2 summarizes selective approaches to nutritional support. The formula 25 kcal/kg + (40 kcal × % body surface area burn) can be used to calculate calorie needs with a 40% or less body surface area burn. Patients with extensive burns (more than 40% of the body) will require an intake above the usual range, up to BEE × 2.0.

Calculating protein needs

The optimal protein intake, like calorie intake, initially can be approximated only and is normally based on the Recommended Dietary Allowance (RDA). The amount of protein recommended for an average healthy adult is 0.8 g/kg/day, but requirements may be increased to 1 to 1.5 g/kg/day in situations of significant physiologic stress with normal renal and hepatic function.

A more precise estimate of protein needs is made on the basis of the 24-hour urine urea nitrogen (UUN) described in Chapter 10. If a patient is receiving little or no protein, a 24-hour UUN gives an estimate of the amount of obligate protein breakdown per day. (UUN g + 4) × 6.25 is an estimate of the daily protein need. An allowance of about 10 g/day above this value is often provided to ensure protein balance.

If the UUN cannot be used, 12% to 16% of total calories as protein can be used as a standard diet for unstressed patients. About 17% to 19% of total calories as protein is an intermediate protein diet; 20% to 25% of calories as protein is a high-protein diet, indicated for highly stressed, hypermetabolic patients and for cachectic patients who are undergoing repletion.

Vitamin and mineral allowances

The best guide to dietary adequacy of vitamins and minerals is the U.S. Recommended Dietary Allowance (RDA) shown in Table 1-1. However, extrapolations must be made for the malnourished or ill patient. Although no guidelines exist for prescribing supplements for patients with illness, Table 10-1 can help identify certain situations in which higher vitamin or mineral allowances should be made.

THERAPEUTIC DIETS

Diet therapy is the most important approach to many disease states, complementing and perhaps even replacing drug therapy in some cases. Therapeutic diets represent permutations of the components of the general diet, which provides optimal health in patients whose condition does not require diet modification.

A useful schema to understand therapeutic diets breaks the general diet into its basic components: water, carbohydrate, protein, fat, vitamins, minerals, and other substances such as alcohol. It is possible to use restrictions or alterations of these components to form a therapeutic diet. For example, a diet may be altered to be low in fat, low in protein, and low in sodium. Certain disease states have commonly prescribed therapeutic diets in which the individual constituents are modified. The following are examples:

- *Water-modified:* restricted fluid intake in severe heart failure, kidney failure.
- *Carbohydrate-modified:* carbohydrate-controlled diet for diabetes and hypertriglyceridemia.
- *Protein-modified:* low protein for the unstressed patient with chronic kidney failure; high protein for the stressed patient.
- *Fat-modified:* low total and saturated fat and low cholesterol for hypercholesterolemia; low total fat for malabsorption syndromes.
- *Vitamin-modified:* restricted vitamin A in renal failure; increased vitamin C in the infected or injured patient.
- *Mineral-modified:* low sodium, potassium, and phosphorus in kidney failure; increased zinc in the infected or injured patient.
- *Other-substances:* restricted alcohol intake for hypertriglyceridemia.

In addition, therapeutic diets may be modified in consistency or texture. Common examples include dental-soft diets for patients without teeth and high-fiber (high-residue) diets for patients with constipation.

Table 11-3   Refeeding after bowel rest

DAY 1

• Clear liquids to check swallowing, followed by low-lactose full liquids (e.g., oral formulas).

DAYS 2-3

• Enteral feeding formula or six small feedings of a low-lactose, soft diet, totaling 30 to 40 g fat per day.
• Buttermilk or *lactobacillus* may be added to reestablish favorable gut flora.

DAYS 4-5

• 50 g fat diet, progressing to regular diet as tolerated.
  Since tube feeding maintains the bowel in a fully functional state, tube-fed patients need not be given this regimen. Rather, their adaptation to oral intake is usually determined by their ability to chew and swallow or by the underlying bowel disease, when present.

Another variation in therapeutic diets involves the sequence in which they are used. The **refeeding diet** is used in patients who have been without enteral feeding for an extended period and who usually have some digestive dysfunction (Table 11-3). The refeeding regimen is a graduated approach to the reintroduction of foods into the diet. The regimen commonly used in the past—going from clear liquid diets to full liquid diets—has two inherent drawbacks: clear liquid diets are high in osmolality and nutritionally inadequate, and full liquid diets are high in fat and lactose. Both of these factors may complicate the refeeding of an impaired intestinal tract. In their place, a lactose-free formula or six small feedings of a low-fat, low-lactose soft diet may be introduced. Buttermilk with active cultures or lactobacillus may be added to reestablish a favorable gut flora if the patient has been taking antibiotics. After several days, the fat content is liberalized and the size of the meals is increased. A regular diet is usually tolerated by the sixth day in patients who have no underlying intestinal disease.

ENTERAL FEEDING

For obvious reasons, oral intake is the preferred method of nutritional support. When this is not possible for more than 3 to 5 days, enteral nutrition, commonly referred to as tube feeding, can be initiated provided the GI tract is functional. Enteral feedings should always be considered before parenteral nutrition because of lower cost, fewer complications, and greater likelihood of maintaining GI mucosal integrity. Its use is widespread in U.S. hospitals and fairly common in the nursing home and home setting.

Feeding approaches

The selection of tubes and pumps specially designed for feeding is quite broad. Because of their pliability and long-term tolerance, small-gauge feeding tubes should virtually always be used for enteral feeding (Fig. 11-3). Because gastric

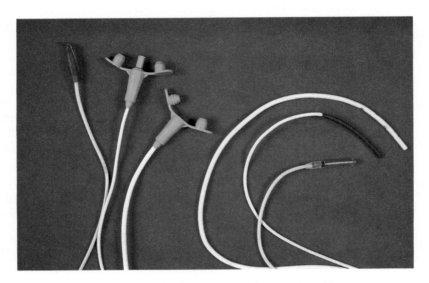

Fig. 11-3   Small-bore feeding tubes used in enteral nutrition support.

contents cannot be reliably aspirated through the soft, small-bore tubes, the need to monitor gastric retention may justify the use of standard large-bore nasogastric tubes in certain patients who are at risk for pulmonary aspiration.

Although soft nasogastric tubes have been used safely for months and even years in some patients, long-term tube feeding is usually best accomplished through a percutaneous endoscopic gastrostomy (PEG). This method of gastrostomy placement in most cases is preferred over surgical gastrostomies because of low morbidity and cost. A PEG tube is placed by passing an endoscope with a light source into the patient's stomach. The light is viewed through the skin and an incision is made, using local anesthesia. The PEG tube is inserted directly through the incision, or directed down the esophagus and out the incision, and secured. Because the risk of pulmonary aspiration is not appreciably lower with gastrostomies than with nasogastric tubes, in patients at high risk for aspiration, duodenal intubation either through the nose or through a PEG is advised.

In patients who are not at high risk for aspiration (i.e., those who are alert and have a normal gag reflex), it is not necessary to confirm tube placement radiographically before beginning feeding. Insufflation of air and auscultation over the stomach and return of bile or gastric contents, followed by monitoring during the first hour of feeding, are usually adequate, and avoid delay of feeding.

Formula selection

The choices of enteral feeding formulas have increased phenomenally in recent years, but formulas often are promoted for features that have little physiological significance. Important criteria for selection of formulas include caloric density, protein content, route of administration, and cost. Caloric density determines the amounts of most nutrients delivered per liter, including not only the calories but also protein, water, and others. Commonly used formulas have a caloric density of 1, 1.5, or 2 kcal/ml. Higher-calorie formulas (1.5 to 2 kcal/ml) can result in dehydration due to inadequate water delivery in patients who are unable to consume additional water ad lib or who have high water requirements. The fluid status of these patients should be carefully monitored. On the other hand, it is not necessary to use commercial starter formulas or diluted standard formulas with a density of 0.5 kcal/ml. The practice of diluting formulas is still somewhat widespread, but there is no evidence that it improves tolerance, and in fact it may increase bacterial contamination of the formula. Feedings should be started at full strength.

When the caloric density has been selected, the formula of choice is usually determined by the protein content, the route of administration (oral or tube), and the lowest cost. Protein content should be considered not in absolute terms but relative to total calories (as percent of total kilocalories). Formulas that provide more than 20% of calories as protein are considered high in protein.

Less important criteria for formula selection include osmolality, nutrient complexity, and content of fat, lactose, minerals, and residue. There is little evidence that osmolality plays an important role in formula tolerance. Lactose-containing formulas should not be used in acutely ill patients because of the common problem of lactase deficiency. Most of the commonly used formulas are now lactose free, which practically eliminates consideration of lactose content as a criterion for selection. The advantages of oligomeric, or elemental, formulas over those with whole proteins (polymeric formulas) are controversial and should be weighed against their higher cost and osmolality.

Virtually all hospitals have discontinued the preparation of blenderized formulas for inpatient use because of higher personnel cost, poorer quality control, and greater potential for clogging of fine-bore feeding tubes.

Tube-feeding methods

Continuous feeding. The continuous drip method with a closed, aseptic system is generally preferred. A pump should always be used to avoid accidental infusions of dangerously large volumes. Continuous feeding assures reliable nutrient delivery and reduces the risks of diarrhea, gastric distention, and pulmonary aspiration of the feeding formula.

The initial infusion rate and the rapidity of its increase should vary, depending on the patient's overall condition. Patients with impaired mental status or prolonged lack of use of the GI tract (>2 weeks) should have feedings introduced and increased more slowly than alert patients whose intestines have been properly functioning recently.

Bolus feeding. This method involves infusing a certain volume of formula into the feeding tube by gravity, over several minutes several times a day. It is most useful for long-term feeding in stable patients and is commonly used in homes and nursing homes. It allows mobility and reduces the cost, since a pump and infusion set are not needed.

Complications

Diarrhea, a common complication of enteral feeding, was once widely thought to be due to the osmolality of feeding solutions. However, there is little evidence for this. The predominant cause for diarrhea associated with tube feeding is probably medications. Diarrhea should not be attributed to enteral feeding until other causes have definitively been ruled out. The following causes should be considered:

- Sorbitol-containing elixirs (acetaminophen, theophylline, and many others). Medication package inserts cannot be relied upon to indicate sorbitol content. Because the content varies among manufacturers, contact with the manufacturer or discontinuation of all enteral medications is often required.
- Magnesium antacids (e.g., Maalox, Mylanta) or other medications.
- Pseudomembranous colitis.
- Bacterial dysentery.

Gastric retention is defined loosely as the presence of more than about 100 ml of gastric contents 2 hours after the last feeding. Although paralytic ileus (the absence of bowel activity) is probably the most common cause, hypokalemia, effects of drugs, and obstruction must be ruled out. Some observers also have reported severe hypoalbuminemia to be a cause of gastric retention. Parenteral feeding is required in cases of unremitting retention.

Pulmonary aspiration of gastric contents is the most feared complication of tube feeding and is the major reason to monitor gastric residual volume. Whenever possible, the patient's head should be elevated during feeding to avoid reflux.

Enteral feeding results in far fewer metabolic complications than does parenteral feeding. The most common complication is probably hyperglycemia, particularly in patients with preexisting glucose intolerance. This can be handled through tighter diabetes control and rarely requires reduction of the feeding.

Tube feeding formulas with high-calorie density or high-protein content do not contain enough water for some patients to handle their renal solute load. Patients on these formulas who are unable to regulate their fluid needs voluntarily and who do not have adequate intravenous fluid intake may become dehydrated, hyperosmolar, and hyperglycemic. The osmolality of the formula is not related to these problems, because carbohydrates (the major osmotic component) are ordinarily metabolized and do not contribute to the renal solute load. The fluid status and blood glucose levels of patients at risk should be closely monitored.

PARENTERAL NUTRITION

Parenteral nutrition, or intravenous feeding, has been referred to as total parenteral nutrition (TPN) and as hyperalimentation (hyperal, or HA). The latter term is not preferred since it implies an excessive amount of nutrients is delivered. It can also be described more specifically as central venous alimentation (CVA) or peripheral venous alimentation (PVA). Several of these terms will be used interchangeably in this section.

With parenteral nutrition, calories are supplied by carbohydrate in the form of dextrose, and fat as vegetable-oil emulsions. Protein is supplied by crystalline amino acids. Vitamins, minerals, and trace elements are added in chemical form. Certain medications, such as insulin, can be added to the TPN solution when necessary.

Indications for parenteral nutrition

Some of the indications for parenteral nutrition include (1) a nonfunctioning GI tract due to conditions such as short bowel syndrome from trauma, infection, or infarction resulting in surgical resection; adynamic ileus from sepsis or other severe illness; or obstruction; (2) conditions in which bowel rest is desirable such as inflammatory bowel disease or intestinal fistulas; (3) certain cases of severe malnutrition prior to surgery. Usually parenteral nutrition is used when oral or enteral intake is inadequate to meet the patient's needs for more than 3 to 5 days.

The contraindications to parenteral nutrition are all relative; there are no situations in which a person should *absolutely* not be fed. Relative contraindications include the presence of a functional GI tract (surprisingly, some clinicians still tend to resort to TPN when enteral feeding could be used), intended use for less than 3 to 5 days, and a patient who will die imminently due to underlying disease. Specific exceptions to these can be cited, so each case should be evaluated on its own merit.

Routes of administration

To attain sufficient calorie intake without giving excessive volumes of fluid, the nonprotein calories must be concentrated. This is achieved by using final concentrations of up to 35% dextrose. It results in a fluid osmolality of roughly 1800 mOsm/kg water, which is very irritating to the venous endothelium. Therefore, these solutions must be infused into central veins, where they are rapidly diluted by high blood-flow rates. Typically, the catheter tip is introduced into the superior vena cava via the subclavian or internal jugular vein (Fig. 11-4).

When central venous catheterization is undesirable or when parenteral nutrition is desired for short periods, more dilute solutions can be infused into peripheral veins. Even with final dextrose concentrations of only 10%, the os-

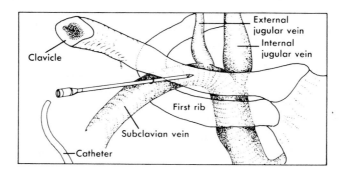

Fig. 11-4 A schematic diagram describing method and location for placement of a subclavian catheter for central venous alimentation.

molality of these formulas is 900 to 1100 mOsm/kg water, resulting in fairly short periods of vein patency due to phlebitis. To meet caloric requirements, intravenous lipid emulsions should be used daily as a source of calories to compensate for the dilute dextrose. Total volumes of more than 3 L/day often must be used, exceeding the tolerance of many patients.

Nonprotein calorie sources

The major source of nonprotein calories in TPN, dextrose (d-glucose), is provided in the monohydrous form, reducing its calorie yield to 3.4 kcal/g rather than the 4 kcal/g in dry (dietary) carbohydrate. Dextrose contributes the majority of the osmolality of the TPN solution. It is supplied by manufacturers in concentrations up to 70%.

Intravenous lipid emulsions are available in 10% (1.1 kcal/ml) or 20% (2 kcal/ml) concentrations derived from safflower oil, soybean oil, or a combination of the two. These emulsions can be given piggy-back at the same time as the TPN solution or mixed with dextrose and amino acids in 3-in-1 admixtures (i.e., protein, carbohydrate, and fat in the same bag) in a variety of concentrations, as long as certain guidelines are observed. The addition of lipids reduces the osmolality and hence the caustic nature of parenteral nutrition (Fig. 11-5).

In CVA, lipid emulsions must be used at least weekly to prevent essential fatty acid (EFA) deficiency. The continuous infusion of concentrated dextrose and the consequent steady elevation of insulin levels can prevent mobilization of endogenous adipose tissue stores of EFA, thereby resulting in biochemical evidence of EFA deficiency within a week. Lipid emulsions prevent this. When a clear contraindication to the use of lipid emulsions exists (and this is extremely

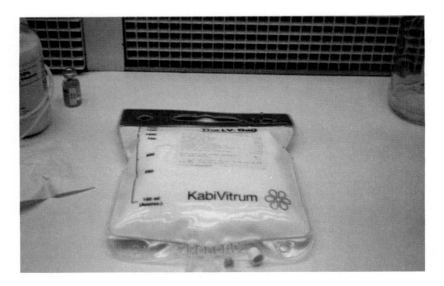

Fig. 11-5   A three-in-one admixture used for central venous alimentation.

rare), topical application of small amounts of a vegetable oil such as safflower oil to the arms or legs twice daily can prevent EFA deficiency but may not be sufficient to correct it if the deficiency is already present. If three-in-one solutions are not used, it is recommended to give lipid continuously to provide a source of calories. Studies have shown daily and continuous administration of lipids to be the most physiologic and beneficial.

In some patient groups, the use of daily lipid calories is particularly beneficial. In diabetic patients, better glucose tolerance and lower insulin requirements can be achieved when less dextrose is infused. Patients with ventilatory failure and CO_2 retention, especially those without hypoxemia, can benefit from the lesser CO_2 production associated with lipid oxidation as opposed to glucose oxidation.

The adverse effects of intravenous lipid emulsions are very few. Severe hypoxemia can be aggravated by rapid infusion of lipid if the clearance of circulating triglycerides is delayed. However, this complication can nearly always be prevented by infusion of the required amount over 24 hours. Significant underlying hypertriglyceridemia (greater than 500 mg/dl), especially when associated with pancreatitis, can represent a contraindication to the use of intravenous lipid. To check for lipid intolerance, a random serum triglyceride level should be checked at some point during the lipid infusion.

Amino acid solutions

Protein is supplied as synthetic crystalline amino acids, which are safe, effective, and widely available in concentrations between 3.5% and 15% (3.5 to 15 g/100 ml). They yield 4 kcal/g. Except in patients who are in markedly positive nitrogen balance, the protein intake is generally assumed to be replacing protein that is oxidized. Thus, the infused protein is contributing to the total calorie consumption and is generally included as part of the total calories of a CVA mixture.

Vitamins

The RDA for micronutrients do not apply to parenteral nutrition because the absorptive process is bypassed. Guidelines for parenteral vitamin requirements have been embodied in the commercial multivitamin preparations most commonly used in TPN. They have been shown to be adequate for the maintenance of vitamin status when it is already normal, but they may not be adequate to correct preexisting vitamin deficiencies or to meet the needs of ill patients with increased requirements. For example, vitamin C requirements are increased in the stress state, so it is often advisable to use added amounts—generally 500 to 1000 mg per day.

Minerals

The major electrolytes provided in parenteral nutrition are sodium, potassium, calcium, magnesium and phosphorus. It is possible to make changes in the patient's mineral and acid-base status by altering the levels of these and the anions chosen for each. For example, by substituting acetate for chloride, with or without changes in sodium and potassium intake, it is possible to help correct significant acidoses. Likewise, when the patient needs more phosphorus, it can be given as the sodium or potassium salt if either cation must be limited.

Trace elements

As in the case of vitamins, multiple trace element solutions are available that satisfy the maintenance requirements of most patients. These usually include zinc, copper, chromium, and manganese. Additional zinc should be used for patients who have increased requirements, such as stressed and postoperative patients, and for those with increased losses such as may result from small-bowel diarrhea.

Iron dextran can be added to parenteral nutrition solutions when needed. However, because most patients are not on TPN long enough for poor intake to deplete their body iron stores, this is rarely necessary. A test dose should be given first when administering iron parenterally because of a small risk of anaphylaxis. Selenium may need to be added for patients on long-term (home) TPN.

Management of parenteral nutrition

The TPN catheter should be placed in the superior vena cava (see Fig. 11-4). Calorie and protein requirements should be calculated as described in Chapter 11. It is often helpful to calculate the protein requirement relative to calories (percent of calories as protein), also discussed in Chapter 11. This helps one choose the relative amounts of amino acids and nonprotein calorie sources to be included in the TPN regimen. One must also decide whether to use intravenous lipid daily or intermittently during the week.

The initial infusion rate varies with different patients. Highly stressed patients who have been receiving intravenous dextrose infusions can be started at about 50 ml/hr and advanced quickly, usually about every 8 to 12 hours, to reach their full calorie requirements within 24 to 48 hours. Severely cachectic, chronically starved, nonstressed patients should be fed at about 0.8 × basal energy expenditure (BEE) the first day and then increased stepwise to 1.5 × BEE over about 7 days (or, if stable, gradually increased to 2 × BEE for weight gain).

Dextrose infusion stimulates insulin secretion that lasts for a short while after cessation of the dextrose flow. Therefore, if termination of the infusion is abrupt, hypoglycemia occasionally ensues. Although many TPN patients are protected from this by stress-induced, insulin-resistant hyperglycemia, it is wise to reduce the infusion rate by 50% to 70% for 30 to 60 minutes before discontinuing parenteral nutrition. This is unnecessary if the patient is being fed enterally or orally when the infusion is discontinued.

Aside from proper general medical and nursing care, careful laboratory monitoring is important during TPN. Alterations in electrolytes and other blood parameters often necessitate adjustment of the parenteral nutrition formula.

Complications

Complications of parenteral nutrition fall into three main categories: technical, infectious, and metabolic. They can nearly always be avoided by careful patient management. Technical complications relate to the placement of a central venous catheter and are therefore not unique to parenteral nutrition. The most common of these is pneumothorax (air introduced into the thorax), which is best prevented by careful, unhurried insertion of the central line by an experienced physician.

Venous thrombosis is another potentially serious complication. Prolonged bed rest, certain malignancies, and hypercoagulable states increase the risk. Low-dose oral warfarin (Coumadin) or heparin added to the TPN solution can decrease the risk of this complication. Infections can be systemic or local. Sepsis, when it occurs in the TPN patient, is usually due to poor technique in aseptic catheter care and is therefore not unique to parenteral nutrition. It can be prevented by standard nursing guidelines and periodic catheter replacement. The offending organisms are usually skin contaminants, but in hospitalized patients gram-negative infections may occur. Definite catheter sepsis may require removal of the catheter, but it can usually be replaced. Site infections can usually be treated with meticulous site care without removal of the catheter.

Metabolic complications remain the most common, since metabolic requirements (e.g., electrolytes, calories) cannot be reduced to standardized guidelines. In our experience, the most serious of these is sudden, severe hypophosphatemia induced by dextrose infusion. Although phosphorus levels drop in most patients after TPN begins, severely cachectic patients are the most susceptible to potentially lethal consequences. It is usually advisable to put phosphorus in the TPN solution of all patients unless a specific contraindication exists. The risk of transient hyperphosphatemia is minimal except in hypercalcemic patients. The serum levels of phosphorus, as well as other electrolytes, should be monitored periodically, especially when initiating TPN. Adjustments in the TPN solution can then be made as required.

The most common, but less serious, metabolic abnormality in TPN patients is hyperglycemia. It is treated by correcting hypophosphatemia if present (a cause of glucose intolerance), adding insulin to the TPN solution, reducing the dextrose load by substituting lipid for dextrose, and ensuring that the total caloric load is not excessive.

Other metabolic complications include hypokalemia and hyperkalemia, which can be prevented and treated by using appropriate amounts of potassium in the TPN. Hyponatremia and hypernatremia require assessment of both sodium and water balance and should be treated by appropriate alterations in total sodium and water intake.

Abnormalities in liver functions occur frequently in patients on parenteral nutrition. The cause is probably fatty deposits in the liver, induced by the constant dextrose infusion. It is usually benign and self-limited, requiring no intervention. If progressive increases in the tests are seen, cycling the TPN, (infusing the same caloric load in a shorter time and giving the liver a rest during part of each day) often is effective. If this is not corrective, causes other than the TPN should be considered.

Home parenteral nutrition

Just as other modalities of therapy such as renal dialysis have been adapted for home use, home TPN enables selected patients who depend on parenteral feeding to return to a reasonably normal life-style. A specialized catheter is introduced

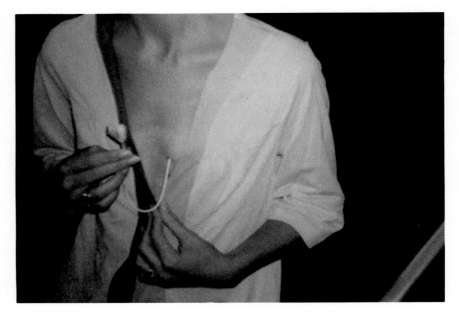

Fig. 11-6   A specialized catheter used for home central venous alimentation.

through a tunnel under the skin to reduce the likelihood of infection. The catheter exits the chest at a place where the patient can care for it conveniently (Fig. 11-6). Infusing the necessary solutions during the night while the patient sleeps leaves him or her free to leave the home and even work during the day. If the intestinal tract is functioning, although inadequately, TPN can be used to supplement oral intake, perhaps by infusing the TPN several nights a week. Home TPN is an expensive investment, but the cost is offset by allowing the patient to leave the hospital sooner and in many cases to resume a productive life-style.

SELECTED READING

Clinical Staff, Dietary Department, University of Iowa Hospitals and Clinics: *Recent advances in therapeutic diets,* ed 4, Ames, Iowa, 1989, Iowa State University Press.

Rombeau JL, Caldwell MD: *Enteral and Tube Feeding,* ed 2, Philadelphia, 1990, WB Saunders.

Rombeau JL, Caldwell MD: *Parenteral Nutrition,* vol 2, Philadelphia, 1986, WB Saunders.

Weinsier RL, Heimburger DC, Butterworth CE Jr: *Handbook of Clinical Nutrition,* ed 2, St. Louis, 1989, CV Mosby.

12

Nutritional Support of Special Medical Problems

Nutrition and renal failure
Nutrition and liver disease
Nutrition and pulmonary disease

NUTRITION AND RENAL FAILURE

The kidneys play a crucial role in maintaining optimal metabolic homeostasis of the body. In addition to important regulatory functions, the kidneys provide synthetic, degradative, and hormonal functions. Therefore, as renal function deteriorates, a wide spectrum of metabolic abnormalities may occur, including

- Impaired regulation of sodium, potassium, phosphorus, magnesium, water, and hydrogen ions
- Impaired clearance of urea and other nitrogenous metabolites
- Impaired vitamin D metabolism
- Altered calcium and phosphorus metabolism
- Decreased synthesis of erythropoietin
- Increased clearance of pyridoxine (vitamin B_6)

The severity of these changes will reflect the duration of renal failure (acute or chronic) and the degree of catabolic stress associated with any underlying disease state. The role of nutritional support in renal failure is to prevent or reverse associated malnutrition, minimize toxicity from inappropriate intake of a wide variety of nutrients, and favorably affect the progression and outcome of renal failure.

Chronic renal failure

A broad spectrum of manifestations and outcomes are associated with chronic renal failure (CRF), correlating with the extent of available functioning nephrons. For example, patients with renal function greater than 50% of normal (i.e., serum creatinine of ≤ 2 mg/dl) may have a stable clinical course with minimal adverse metabolic sequelae and minimal need for metabolic and nutritional interventions. The emphasis in such patients should be to maintain optimal nutritional status and prevent further renal deterioration.

For patients with 20% to 50% of normal renal function (that is, serum creatinine between 2 and 5 mg/dl), mild anemia and retention of sodium, potassium, magnesium, phosphorus, and water, nutritional regulation becomes

161

paramount. With progressive CRF there is increasing evidence of wasting and malnutrition as seen by a decrease in fat and lean body compartments, diminished protein synthesis including albumin, and reduced growth rates in children. With appropriate nutritional modifications especially protein, the progression of CRF may be substantially reduced and stabilized and dialysis possibly delayed.

Finally, patients with renal function less than 20% of normal (that is, serum creatinine >5 mg/dl with a blood urea nitrogen greater than 100) are likely to require dialysis, because nutritional regulation only, at this point, may not be sufficient to control uremic symptoms. In this instance, dialysis is an adjunct to continuing restricted nutritional intake, especially protein. However, with the addition of dialysis, these nutritional restrictions may be somewhat liberalized.

Acute renal failure

Acute renal failure (ARF) involves an abrupt and marked decrease in the glomerular filtration rate due to a wide variety of insults to the kidney such as infection, exogenous nephrotoxins, trauma, dehydration, and shock. Urine output is reduced (oliguria) or halted (anuria). As previously noted, fluid and electrolyte balance becomes rapidly deranged because of failure of regulation. The patient with ARF is often highly catabolic because of the associated stress of the underlying disease state. With the advent of dialysis, a patient with ARF can be well supported, minimizing fluid and electrolyte abnormalities and reducing uremic symptoms. However, the ravages of catabolism, including poor wound healing, increased infections, and increased mortality, are unaffected by dialysis alone. Appropriately aggressive nutritional support is strongly indicated. In fact, it is the availability of dialysis adjunctively that allows full nutritional support without regard to the buildup of toxic metabolic products.

Nutritional support of renal failure

Ideally, a patient's nutritional needs are met by oral intake. However, if the patient is unable to accomplish this because of disability or because nutrient demands exceed the patient's ability to maintain adequate intake, enteral or total parenteral nutritional support is indicated. If the gastrointestinal (GI) tract is fully functional, then enteral feeding is preferred. However, the greater the catabolic stress associated with the underlying illness in renal failure, the less likely is the GI tract to absorb nutrients. In this case, total parenteral nutrition may be indicated and can be used exclusively or in combination with enteral feeding.

Energy requirements

The number of kilocalories required is a function of basal energy expenditure (BEE) and the level of associated catabolic stress (if any). An unstressed patient will require approximately 1.2 × BEE kcals/day. However, a hypermetabolic patient may well require 1.2 to 1.5 × BEE kcals/day, depending on the estimated level of stress.

Protein requirements

Provision of adequate but not excessive protein is crucial to the nutritional management of renal failure, especially for the predialysis phase of CRF. For such patients, the appropriate level of daily protein intake may be estimated from the level of glomerular filtration rate (GFR) as follows: 20 to 25 ml/min, 60 to 90 g; 15 to 20 ml/min, 50 to 60 g; 10 to 15 ml per minute, 40 to 50 g. For a GFR of 4 to 10 ml/min approximately 0.55 to 0.60 g/kg/day is indicated. High levels of biological protein are necessary to provide enough essential amino acids for synthesis. These recommendations can stabilize the blood urea nitrogen (BUN) at less than 90 mg/dl in otherwise stable renal-failure patients and thereby control the progression of uremic symptoms. The use of supplementary ketoacid analogs of amino acids is under investigation and holds promise to provide even more effective control of BUN levels and uremic symptoms.

If the GFR is less than 4 to 5 ml/minute, dialysis will be needed. Patients who require maintenance hemodialysis will require 1 to 1.2 g/kg/day of protein. Those receiving peritoneal dialysis will require 1.2 to 1.5 g/kg/day of protein.

High biological value protein sources (i.e., animal sources) are recommended, but they can be combined with lower biological value proteins from vegetable sources. A balanced mixture of essential and nonessential amino acids is recommended for both enteral and parenteral formulas.

Special renal amino acid formulas that contain mainly essential amino acids have limited indications and are for short-term use only. For example, they may be indicated for a brief period where dialysis is delayed because of logistical problems. The use of these formulas on a long-term basis is inappropriate.

Lipid intake

Elevation of triglycerides and diminished levels of high-density lipoprotein cholesterol can be seen in patients with predialysis CRF as well as in those undergoing maintenance hemodialysis. Dietary changes may be necessary to control these abnormalities. When patients receive fat emulsions as part of total parenteral nutrition infusion, it is important to monitor serum triglyceride levels at first to identify hypertriglyceridemia.

Vitamins

CRF patients may be deficient in water-soluble vitamins as a result of poor oral intake and/or losses from dialysis. Pyridoxine (vitamin B_6) has an increased clearance as already noted. Therefore, patients with predialysis CRF should receive the Recommended Dietary Allowance of all water-soluble vitamins in addition to daily administration of the following:

- Folic acid: 1 mg
- Vitamin C: 70 to 100 mg
- Pyridoxine (vitamin B_6): 5 mg

For patients receiving dialysis, these recommendations should be expanded to include at least 100 mg of vitamin C and 10 mg of pyridoxine.

Vitamin requirements in ARF are probably qualitatively similar to those in

CRF. However, it may be that the increased catabolic rate associated with ARF produces an increased turnover of water-soluble vitamins and an increased demand for their replacement. From a clinical standpoint, it is reasonable to obtain baseline vitamin levels and appropriate follow-up.

Vitamin D deficiency occurs in CRF because of the inability of the kidney to form 1,25-dihydroxycholecalciferol, which is the activated form of vitamin D, from 25-hydroxycholecalciferol. Vitamin D replacement is indicated if vitamin D deficiency is present. However, to avoid the formation of calcium phosphate precipitates in soft tissue, it is important that vitamin D not be started if either calcium or phosphorus is elevated.

Vitamin A levels may be elevated in renal failure because of the inability to excrete retinol-binding protein. Therefore, vitamin A supplementation in these patients should be avoided unless there is a clear, documented indication to do so clinically.

Fluid and electrolytes

Sodium and water. Sodium and water balance may be abnormal in CRF. In some instances, excessive retention of sodium and water occurs and predisposes to edema, hypertension, and congestive heart failure. In other instances, the kidney may not be able to retain sodium and water, which predisposes to dehydration, hypotension, and further reduction in renal function as a result of reduced GFR. Because the former circumstance is more common, restriction of sodium and water intake usually is appropriate, depending on the level of renal failure and on the amount of urine output. An appropriate starting point for daily restriction would be 1 to 3 g of sodium and a fluid intake sufficient to exceed urine output by 500 ml (to cover insensible water losses). Adjustments to this can be made according to the clinical response to the restrictions. The goal is to establish optimal body water, normalize blood pressure and serum sodium, and eliminate edema. Frequent weighing helps to monitor daily shifts of body water.

Potassium. The kidney is the primary route of potassium excretion. Therefore, potassium restriction to 40 to 60 mEq/day is appropriate in renal failure. It is important to be alert to increases in potassium levels in acidosis, oliguria, and increasing catabolism.

Phosphorus. The kidney is also responsible for phosphorus excretion. Elevation of serum phosphorus leads to a depression of serum calcium, which in turn stimulates parathyroid hormone release and eventually leads to hyperparathyroidism. It is possible that hyperphosphatemia and/or hyperparathyroidism may have a link to progressive renal failure. Therefore, it is important to keep serum phosphorus at the lower range of normal by reducing intake to the range of 600 to 1200 mg/day and by the use of phosphate binders such as aluminum hydroxide.

Calcium. CRF patients have reduced intestinal calcium absorption that is related to abnormal vitamin D metabolism as noted. Therefore, CRF patients should receive 1000 to 1500 mg/day of supplemental calcium. It is important to initiate calcium supplementation only after serum phosphorus is normalized.

Magnesium. Normally magnesium is excreted by the kidney. Therefore, magnesium is often restricted to approximately 200 mg/day in CRF patients. Magnesium-containing medications, such as certain antacids and laxatives, should be discontinued.

Iron. Iron deficiency is common in renal failure and is due to impaired iron absorption in the intestine, occult GI bleeding, blood loss from frequent blood sampling for laboratory studies, and/or sequestration of blood during hemodialysis. Therefore, if needed, 325 mg of ferrous sulfate should be given up to three times per day or in a regimen that is best tolerated by the patient.

pH: Metabolic acidosis may be present in CRF patients because of retention of acids and/or the renal loss of bicarbonate. Calcium carbonate may be useful for mild acidosis. However, sodium bicarbonate given orally or intravenously may be necessary for severe acidosis. Dialysis is indicated if these measures are ineffective in controlling the acidosis.

NUTRITION AND LIVER DISEASE

The liver is the conductor and orchestrator of a wide variety of significant metabolic processes including carbohydrate, fat, and protein metabolism, vitamin storage and activation, and detoxification and excretion of both endogenous and exogenous waste products. Understandably, impaired liver function can produce major imbalances of metabolic and nutritional status. Conversely, progressive impairment of nutritional status can further impair liver function.

Because the liver has an enormous functional reserve (it can perform satisfactorily with only 20% of functioning liver cells and has a marvelous potential to regenerate after injury), the goal of nutritional therapy is to support liver function and to enhance the liver's ability to regenerate after the stress of injury.

Carbohydrate metabolism in liver disease

The liver plays a central role in blood glucose homeostasis. Whenever exogenous sources of glucose are insufficient for the body's requirements, the liver initially increases blood glucose levels by breaking down glycogen. As glycogen stores become depleted, the liver increases glucose availability through the process of gluconeogenesis. With severe hepatic insufficiency, glycogen metabolism and gluconeogenesis may be impaired to the point of causing hypoglycemia.

Fat metabolism in liver disease

The liver plays an important role in normal fat metabolism. Fatty acids from both endogenous and exogenous sources are converted by the liver to acetyl CoA, which is processed by the citric acid cycle for further energy production. As an adaptation to starvation, the liver can form ketone bodies, which can be used by the body, including the brain, as a fuel source in the absence of glucose. This has its advantages as a gluconeogenesis-sparing process that conserves further breakdown of muscle protein sources to form glucose as an energy substrate. Thus, lean body mass is conserved by using ketone bodies rather than glucose as a fuel source. Finally, the liver is involved in cholesterol, bile acid, and lipoprotein synthesis.

As a result of hepatic injury, all of the above functions may be impaired. Fat malabsorption may result from diminished bile salt production and may be associated with fat-soluble vitamin deficiencies.

Protein metabolism and liver disease

As with carbohydrate and fat metabolism, the liver processes both endogenous and exogenous sources of protein. Endogenous proteins are continuously being hydrolyzed and resynthesized. Through transamination, amination, and deamination reactions, there is a constant interchange of amino acid substrates and the substrates of carbohydrate and fat metabolism for the eventual production of energy. Ammonia, a by-product of amino acid metabolism, is converted to urea by the liver and is eventually excreted through the urine.

Altered protein metabolism is probably the most significant consequence of liver disease. It is manifested clinically by encephalopathy and muscle wasting and is characterized by altered plasma amino acid profiles. Typically, the branched-chain amino acids (leucine, isoleucine, and valine) are decreased and the aromatic amino acids (phenylalanine, tyrosine, and tryptophan) and methionine are increased. The precise mechanisms for the development of encephalopathy are complex and multifactorial and relate to the buildup of abnormal amounts of metabolites that interfere with the physiological function of the nervous system. That is, there may be direct interference with neurotransmitter production and function because of the presence of these metabolites and/or possible interference with cerebral energy production.

As hepatic insufficiency develops, the liver becomes less efficient at providing the body with available glucose substrate for energy. As a consequence, the branched-chain amino acids (BCAA) are used locally by several tissue sites as energy substrate. Thus, the BCAA levels decrease. On the other hand, the aromatic amino acids (AAA) are not metabolized normally by the liver, and their levels increase. Since there is competition between the BCAA and the AAA for entry into the brain, with hepatic insufficiency the ratio of AAA/BCAA is increased and more AAA cross the blood-brain barrier. The AAA are the precursors of central neurotransmitters, including the inhibitory neurotransmitter serotonin, and false neurotransmitters. Thus, the inhibition of brain function (i.e., stupor) seems to occur with increasing levels of AAA entering the brain.

Vitamin and trace element metabolism and liver disease

Because the liver is involved in the storage and activation of many vitamins and synthesizes the carrier proteins involved for many of the vitamins, disturbances in vitamin metabolism are present in hepatic insufficiency. The reasons for deficiency include poor oral intake, increased needs associated with the increasing catabolic stresses underlying hepatic insufficiency, and decreased liver storage. By similar mechanisms, there is also impaired metabolism of zinc, copper, potassium, magnesium, molybdenum, cadmium, and selenium.

Treatment of liver disease

Hepatic insufficiency creates a treatment dilemma for the clinician. On one hand, protein intolerance manifested clinically as encephalopathy may occur with even normal amounts of protein intake. On the other hand, protein insufficiency will produce inadequate protein synthesis and result in significant reduction in function of all organ systems, especially the immune and host-defense systems. Therefore, the therapeutic strategy for hepatic insufficiency is to provide both the estimated energy requirements and sufficient protein to establish nitrogen balance without precipitating or exacerbating encephalopathy.

Keeping these principles in mind, the following guidelines may be used to formulate nutritional support:

- As part of the nutritional assessment (see Chapter 10), the 24-hour urinary urea nitrogen is used to determine the appropriate level of protein intake while providing an estimate of the degree of catabolism related to the underlying disease states.
- Fluid and sodium restriction is instituted in the presence of ascites and/ or edema.
- Standard sources of protein for diet replacement and standard fixed formulas for enteral and/or parenteral support are used at first. If the patient has a history of protein intolerance or has encephalopathy, protein delivery should begin at a reduced rate, 0.5 to 0.7 g/kg/day. Thereafter, this can be increased by approximately 10 to 15 g/day in order to precisely determine protein tolerance. If nitrogen balance cannot be achieved with standard formulations because of encephalopathy, then the use of enriched BCAA formulations, either enterally or parenterally, should be considered. The BCAA are useful in achieving nitrogen balance while decreasing the potential for encephalopathy. However, their usefulness in improving outcome in hepatic insufficiency is being studied.
- Dietary fat restriction is unnecessary unless fat malabsorption is present.
- Vitamin and mineral replacement therapy should be initiated and monitored periodically.
- Electrolyte disturbances are treated specifically as they are encountered.
- Finally, it is imperative that periodic nutritional reassessment be done in order to evaluate the therapeutic effectiveness of the support plan.

NUTRITION AND PULMONARY DISEASE

Nutritional status is an important consideration in the assessment and management of chronic obstructive pulmonary disease (COPD) and acute respiratory failure. In patients with previously normal pulmonary function who develop respiratory failure, and especially in patients with acute respiratory failure superimposed on underlying COPD, the risk for developing or exacerbating malnutrition is high. Conversely, malnutrition can affect respiratory muscle function and ventilatory drive. The content of the diet also has an effect on ventilation and gas exchange. Thus, knowledge and application of nutritional principles bear directly on the management and outcome of COPD and respiratory failure.

Patients with COPD, especially emphysema, have an increased likelihood of malnutrition reflected by a reduction in weight, fat reserves, and muscle mass, including the diaphragm and other muscles of respiration (Fig. 12-1). This results from a combination of reduced calorie intake and greater energy demands because of increased work of breathing.

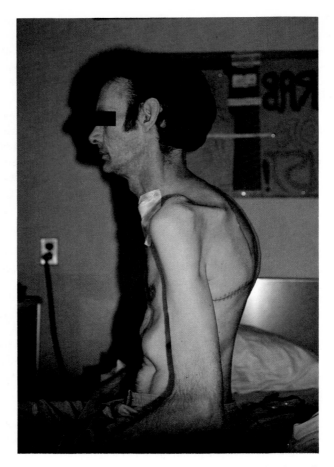

Fig. 12-1   Cachexia in a patient with chronic obstructive lung disease.

The greater the severity of COPD, the greater the associated malnutrition and weight loss; the greater the weight loss, the smaller the weight of the respiratory muscles and the diaphragm. Thus, malnutrition is associated with loss of strength, which contributes to further impairment of respiratory function.

Nutrition and acute respiratory failure

Malnutrition occurs in almost 50% of patients with acute respiratory failure. Whether or not underlying COPD is present, the effects of semistarvation and malnutrition may be taking place. That is, decrease in respiratory muscle structure and function creates decreased muscle strength and easy muscle fatigue. In addition, there is a decrease in ventilatory drive in response to hypoxia and hypercarbia (increased carbon dioxide [CO_2] content of the blood). These factors impair recovery from acute respiratory failure and prolong weaning from mechanical ventilation.

Impairment of the immune system is another adverse effect of malnutrition in respiratory failure. Malnutrition is associated with decreased cell-mediated immunity, altered immunoglobulin production, impaired cellular resistance of the tracheobronchial mucosa to bacterial infection, and possibly a defect in alveolar macrophage function. All of these factors increase the risk of associated infection, especially pneumonia.

Patients with respiratory failure seem especially predisposed to hypophosphatemia. Hypophosphatemia frequently occurs with glucose infusions and causes decreased 2,3-diphosphoglycerate (2,3-DPG) in red blood cells and diminished levels of adenosine triphosphate (ATP). Decreased 2,3-DPG can decrease oxygen delivery to tissues, and decreased ATP production causes impaired respiratory muscle function. Therefore, careful attention must be paid to phosphate status.

Management of respiratory insufficiency

Respiratory insufficiency is characterized by abnormal gas exchange—that is, decreased oxygenation and/or an accumulation of carbon dioxide. The caloric content and nutrient composition of the diet have a profound effect on gas exchange, especially the handling of CO_2.

The respiratory quotient (RQ) is the volume of CO_2 produced divided by the volume of oxygen (O_2) consumed during respiration. The RQ resulting from the oxidation of pure carbohydrate is 1; for fat it is 0.7; and for protein it is 0.8. Thus, more CO_2 is produced by the metabolism of carbohydrate than by the metabolism of fat or protein. A diet composed of relatively few carbohydrate calories and more fat calories produces less CO_2 metabolically. This reduced burden of CO_2 is beneficial for the patient with respiratory insufficiency who may have difficulty exhaling CO_2. On the other hand, a high-carbohydrate diet generates relatively greater amounts of CO_2 and may precipitate frank respiratory failure or increase the difficulty of weaning a patient with respiratory compromise from ventilatory support. Excessive calorie intake as carbohydrate, whether taken orally, enterally, or parenterally, increases the metabolic rate and O_2 requirements and causes even greater CO_2 production. Thus, excessive caloric intake should be avoided.

Previous data have suggested that intravenous infusions of lipid may impair O_2 diffusion capacity across the alveolar capillary bed. This has generally proved to be of no significance in the clinical setting of respiratory insufficiency; nevertheless, the clinician needs to be aware of this potential complicating factor with lipid infusions and monitor patients carefully.

In summary, consider the following in the patient with respiratory compromise:

- Perform a complete nutritional assessment (see Chapter 10).
- Establish appropriate energy and protein needs based on basal energy expenditure and current level of stress. Intake may need to be increased to promote weight gain in the patient with COPD who is not acutely stressed and is metabolically stable. However, intake should not exceed estimated needs in the patient with acute respiratory failure.

- For hypoxic patients, consider reducing the percent of fat calories and proportionately increasing the percent of carbohydrate calories.
- For hypercarbic patients and those being weaned from a respirator, consider reducing the percent of carbohydrate calories and proportionately increasing the percent of fat calories.

Because malnutrition and the mode of refeeding clearly affect outcome in respiratory failure, nutritional therapy is important in both inpatient and outpatient settings. This is especially true when prolonged mechanical ventilation is required. The presence of respiratory failure superimposed on COPD strongly underscores the importance of having a high index of suspicion for malnutrition because a significant proportion of such patients indeed have clinically relevant malnutrition.

Nutritional support can significantly reverse many of the metabolic, biochemical, and physiological alterations found in respiratory insufficiency.

SELECTED READING

Nutrition and renal failure

Maschio G, Oldrizzi L, Rugiu C, et al: Effect of dietary malnutrition of the lipid abnormalities in patients with chronic renal failure, *Kidney Int Suppl* 31, 570-572, 1991.
Protein restriction and the progress of renal insufficiency, *Nutri Rev* 48(8):320-323, 1990.

Nutrition and liver disease

Latifi R, Killam RW, Dudrick SJ: Nutritional support in liver failure, *Surg Clin North Am* 71(3):567-578, 1991.

Nutrition and pulmonary disease

Askanazi J, Nordenstrom J, Rosenbaum SH, et al: Nutrition for the patient with respiratory failure, *Anesthesiology* 54(5):373-377, 1981.
Donahoe M, Rogers RM: Nutrition assessment and support in chronic obstructive pulmonary disease, *Clin Chest Med* 11(3):487-504, 1990.
Fuenzalida CE, Petty TL, Jones ML, et al: The immune response to short-term nutritional intervention in advanced chronic obstructive pulmonary disease, *Am Rev Respir Dis* 142(1):49-56.
Pingleton SK: Nutritional support in the mechanically ventilated patient, *Clin Chest Med* 9(1):101-112, 1988.
Pingleton SK, Harmon GS: Nutritional management in acute respiratory failure, JAMA 257(22):3094-3099, 1987.
Wilson DO, Donahoe M, Rogers RM, Pennock BE: Metabolic rate and weight loss in chronic obstructive lung disease, *JPEN* 14(1):7-11, 1990.
Schwartz J, Weiss ST: Dietary factors and their relation to respiratory symptoms. The Second National Health and Nutrition Examination Survey, *Am J Epidemiol* 132(1):67-76, 1990.

13

Case Studies

Protein-Calorie Malnutrition

Decide whether the numbered statements refer to patient A, patient B, both, or neither.

Patient A is a 52-year-old woman with a 4-year history of weight loss and fatty stools. She formerly weighed 56 kg but now weighs 53 kg and is 165 cm tall. After a "normal" meal she frequently experiences cramping and greasy, foul-smelling stools. She denies having fever, bloody stools, or other complicating illnesses. She has been admitted to the hospital and has had minimal food intake over the past several days (Fig. 13-1A).

Patient B is a 68-year-old male smoker with previously stable chronic lung disease and bronchitis. He has no history of weight loss or significant illness. Prior to admission he had sudden onset of fever, chills, and respiratory failure, which necessitated hospitalization and mechanical ventilatory support. His problems include septic shock (circulatory collapse due to severe infection) and respiratory failure. His weight is 63 kg; his height is 175 cm. He has been in the hospital for 2 weeks without appreciable nutrient intake (Fig. 13-1B).

He or she is
1. Likely to have a reduced metabolic rate (resting energy expenditure).
2. Likely to excrete 15 g urinary urea nitrogen/day (normal, <5g with recent low intake of protein).
3. Likely to have marked elevation of circulating epinephrine.
4. Likely to excrete less than 600 mg creatinine per day in the urine (normal 800 to 1800 mg).
5. Likely to have a serum albumin level of 1.8 g/dl (normal >3.5).
6. Likely to have a triceps skinfold measurement at 20% of standard.
7. Probably relatively well adapted to the energy-deprived state.
8. Particularly susceptible to heart failure upon refeeding with carbohydrate.

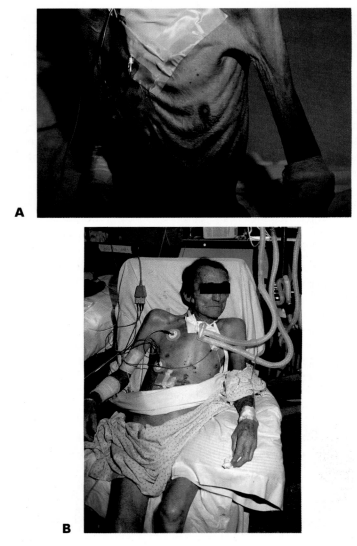

Fig. 13-1   A, Patient A: history of weight loss. **B,** Patient B: history of respiratory failure.

CASE
STUDY **6** *Nutrition Assessment and Support*

A 63-year-old woman was hospitalized for therapy of cervical cancer. She consumed a diet consisting primarily of cornbread, grits, mustard greens (cooked by boiling for several hours), and cereals. She denied eating fresh fruit or vegetables, and she had no teeth. Her appetite was poor and her weight fell from 54 kg to 47 kg over the past 2 months. She ate relatively little in the hospital and was maintained only on intravenous saline solutions. Five days after undergoing total pelvic exenteration (removal of lower abdominal organs as treatment for the cancer), she was noted to have bloody fluid leaking from an evidently poorly healing surgical wound (Fig. 13-2).

Physical examination: There was easy and painless hair pluckability. There were perifollicular petechiae (pinpoint hemorrhages around hair follicles) over the lower extremities, large areas of bleeding into the skin at needle puncture sites, and widespread pitting edema. Her temperature was elevated at 39.5°C. Weight was 63 kg, height 150 cm (reference ideal weight is 47 kg).

Laboratory data: She had a severely reduced lymphocyte count (120 cells/mm^3), blood urea nitrogen (BUN) of 6 mg/dl and serum albumin 2 g/dl; 24-hour urine urea nitrogen excretion was 16 g.

TRUE or FALSE:

1. On oral examination, you would be likely to find swollen, bleeding gums.
2. She has a clear case of kwashiorkor.
3. She is most likely obese.

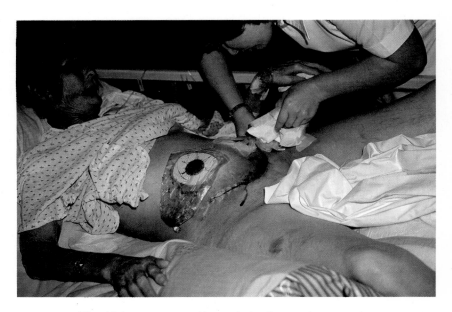

Fig. 13-2 A woman with poorly healing surgical wounds.

4. The low BUN in this case suggests that her recent intake of protein was relatively low and possibly inadequate.
5. A reasonable estimate of her protein needs (i.e., amount needed to be in protein balance) is 185 g/day.
6. Glucose is the only endogenously produced fuel that can be used by this patient's damaged, unoxygenated tissues.

Due to poor oral intake of food and gastric retention on nasogastric tube feeding, central venous alimentation was instituted. The regimen included 500 g dextrose, 100 g protein, 2.5 mg zinc, and routine amounts of electrolytes and vitamins infused continuously over each 24-hour period.

TRUE or FALSE:
7. The glucose content of the parenteral alimentation fluids will effectively decrease protein breakdown to a basal (nonstress) level.
8. An intravenous source of essential fatty acids will not be required in this case, even if none are taken by mouth, because her fat reserves should adequately supply her needs for a number of months.
9. She will be receiving 1700 kcal/day from dextrose.
10. She should be given a larger amount of zinc.

(See appendix for answers and discussion.)

APPENDICES

APPENDIX

A

CASE STUDIES—ANSWERS

Case Study 1: Obesity
Case Study 2: Hyperlipidemia and diabetes
Case Study 3: Alcohol and nutrient deficiencies
Case Study 4: Malabsorption syndrome
Case Study 5: Protein-calorie malnutrition
Case Study 6: Nutrition assessment and support

CASE STUDY 1 *Obesity*

1. *False*. Blood cholesterol levels tend to be only slightly higher in obese than in normal-weight people when diet and other factors are controlled. The elevated cholesterol in this case is more likely secondary to the high-fat, carbohydrate-restricted diet that has been reported to increase low-density lipoprotein and total cholesterol levels.

2. *True*. Carbohydrate-restricted diets frequently produce ketosis with ketone excretion in the urine. Because there is competition for excretion of ketones and uric acid, the presence of ketones in the urine will increase uric acid retention and produce elevated blood uric acid levels.

3. *True*. It is well established that the presence of obesity increases the likelihood that an otherwise predisposed individual will develop diabetes. However, if diabetes is not present, ingestion of a carbohydrate-restricted diet will quickly result in glucose intolerance (equivalent to "starvation diabetes"), possibly giving a false impression of the presence of diabetes.

4. *False*. Ketones in the urine will appear after a several-day fast, but the most likely explanation here is inadequate carbohydrate intake that mimics starvation ketosis. Ketosis clears quickly with reintroduction of carbohydrates (starches, fruits, or sugars).

5. *False*. Restriction of all carbohydrates is rarely, if ever, indicated for a person with diabetes, especially since this results in a high intake of fats and its associated increased risk for coronary artery disease. Selected carbohydrates, especially simple sugars, may need to be restricted, or the carbohydrates should be distributed more evenly throughout the day; however, total carbohydrate intake is generally prescribed at about 50% of total calories to keep the fat intake down.

CASE
STUDY **2** *Hyperlipidemia and Diabetes*

1. *True*. The creamy layer over the serum observed after allowing the blood to stand indicates that chylomicrons are present in the circulation. When there is a high concentration, as in this case, a creamy appearance will be evident in the retinal vessels (lipemia retinalis).

2. *False*. Because of its association with coronary artery disease, low-density lipoprotein cholesterol is the lipid of greatest concern; and its level is usually proportional to the total cholesterol level. However, when triglyceride levels are notably increased, as in this case, a certain proportion of the total cholesterol will be carried in the chylomicrons and the very low-density lipoprotein (pre-β lipoprotein) fractions. Thus, without further laboratory analyses, it would be impossible to say that low-density lipoprotein cholesterol was abnormal in this case.

3. *False*. Although the presence of juvenile-onset, insulin-dependent diabetes is associated with the type I pattern of hyperlipoproteinemia, this patient appears to have type 5 hyperlipoproteinemia. Hyperchylomicronemia is seen in both types I and V, but increased very low-density lipoprotein (giving turbidity to the serum as in this case) goes along with the type V pattern.

4. *False*. In contrast to the tendinous and tuberous xanthomas observed most often in the type II pattern (increased low-density lipoprotein cholesterol), which are more often associated with the true genetic form, the eruptive xanthomas of the skin (in this case) can appear and disappear in a relatively short time. This is related to the degree of elevation of triglycerides and is often not associated with a genetic disorder.

5. *False*. In this case, the abnormal lipid pattern is probably due to the uncontrolled diabetes. With improved control of the diabetes, it can be expected that the lipid levels will improve markedly. No decision about drug therapy for the lipid abnormality should be made at this time.

6. *True*. The use of certain types of fiber and fiber-containing foods has been found to be associated with improved blood sugar and insulin levels and even to reduce insulin requirements.

7. *False*. Increased alcohol intake has been associated with increased high-density lipoprotein cholesterol; however, it has not been recommended for nondrinkers for the purpose of elevating high-density lipoprotein cholesterol. Alcohol intake should be kept to a minimum in people with a type V pattern of hyperlipidemia.

CASE
STUDY **3** *Alcohol and Nutrient Deficiencies*

1. *False*. Hypersegmented neutrophils are not associated with vitamin C deficiency but are a classic manifestation of folate or vitamin B_{12} deficiency.

2. *False*. The RDA for riboflavin for this person is 1.6 mg/day. His riboflavin intake from milk alone will be at least this amount.

3. *True*. Alcohol is known to decrease the absorption of thiamin. Ethanol intake of 1.5 to 2 g/kg body weight has been shown to decrease absorption by 40%.

4. *False*. Although there is some evidence to suggest a decrease in the production of intrinsic factor and hence a decrease in B_{12} absorption with alcohol intake, the clinical relevance is unclear. The more likely explanation for these hematologic abnormalities is folate deficiency, which is not uncommonly seen in alcoholism (up to 90%) due to poor intake and impaired absorption and utilization.

5. *True*. The history of alcohol abuse, the poor dietary intake, the use of antacids (which decrease thiamin absorption), and the clinical manifestations of Korsakoff's psychosis, ataxia, weakness, and peripheral neuropathy are all compatible with thiamin deficiency.

6. *False*. Although there is increased risk of pellagra in the alcoholic, this is still uncommonly seen in the United States, and this patient has no clinical manifestations of pellagra (recall the four Ds: dementia, diarrhea, dermatitis, and death).

7. *False*. Although alcoholics may have increased iron loss from bleeding, iron deficiency is not often seen in this group because of increased absorption of iron, bone-marrow suppression (reducing requirements), and the presence of iron in certain alcoholic beverages such as red wine. In this patient, there is no clinical evidence of iron deficiency such as microcytic (small-celled) anemia; the slick tongue that occurs as a result of iron deficiency may be seen rarely, but it is more likely due to folate deficiency in this case.

8. *False*. His diet is certainly low in vitamin C; however, without laboratory documentation or clinical evidence of scurvy such as unemerged coiled hairs, perifollicular petechiae, gum changes and so on, it would be impossible to make the diagnosis.

9. *False*. Renal excretion of zinc is increased by alcohol intake, and zinc deficiency is more common in the alcoholic. However, without laboratory confirmation or clinical manifestations such as altered sense of taste or smell, dry scaly skin, or reduced wound healing, the diagnosis cannot be confirmed.

CASE
STUDY **4**   *Malabsorption Syndrome*

1. *False*. Normally, a low serum carotene level is indicative of a poor intake of green and yellow-orange fruits and vegetables (sources of carotene, the provitamin form of vitamin A). On the other hand, in the presence of fat malabsorption, a low serum carotene level would be expected regardless of the intake.

2. *False*. Even in cases of significant fat malabsorption, vitamin C intake and absorption are often adequate. Intake in this case appears to be good, and there is no clear evidence of vitamin C deficiency. Bleeding into the skin is not a finding specific for vitamin C deficiency, in contrast to perifollicular petechiae (pinpoint hemorrhages around hair follicles).

3. *True*. In light of this history, which is compatible with fat malabsorption, this patient has an increased risk of fat-soluble vitamin deficiency, including vitamin K. In most instances, however, vitamin K deficiency does not actually develop, because vitamin K is still produced by the flora of the large intestine. In this case, use of oral antibiotics may have suppressed the intestinal flora, thereby decreasing vitamin K production; and with poor absorption this may have resulted in vitamin K deficiency and its associated bleeding into the skin.

4. *True*. In a person with fat malabsorption, free fatty acids can be expected to be released from dietary fat (triglycerides) through the action of pancreatic lipase. However, without adequate small-bowel function for absorption of the free fatty acids, there will be binding of the fatty acids with divalent cations (including calcium, magnesium, and zinc) and loss of these minerals as soaps in the stool.

5. *True*. In fat malabsorption and short-bowel syndromes, oxalate absorption is increased. This may be explained in part by increased efficiency of absorption in patients with shortened small bowel and in part by the unavailability of calcium for precipitation of oxalate in the bowel (since calcium is now bound to fatty acids). The increased oxalate absorption results in increased excretion and risk of kidney stones.

6. *False*. The terminal ileum is required for the absorption of the intrinsic factor-bound vitamin B_{12}. In the absence of the terminal ileum, B_{12} should be given by injection to prevent a deficiency that may otherwise develop over the course of 2 or 3 years.

CASE
STUDY **5**   *Protein-Calorie Malnutrition*

1. *Patient A*. The patient evidently has malabsorption, severe weight loss, and cachexia (chronic starvation). In this situation and in the absence of acute stress, the metabolic rate is reduced as the body attempts to conserve energy. By contrast, patient B will be hypermetabolic due to the septic state.

2. *Patient B*. The rate of urea nitrogen excretion is proportional to the degree of gluconeogenesis as the body breaks down protein in an attempt to produce glucose in response to the stressed state. This certainly applies to patient B, whereas patient A is semistarved and will be expected to have a relatively low rate of gluconeogenesis.

3. *Patient B*. Circulating catecholamines and urinary catecholmines tend to be elevated in the presence of acute stress such as that from sepsis or trauma. This is part of the fight or flight response.

4. *Patient A*. Urinary creatinine excretion is generally proportional to one's muscle mass, because creatinine is formed from creatine, which is derived from the muscle.

5. *Patient B*. An albumin level of 1.8 g/dl is significantly reduced and in the case of patient B is a reflection of the severely stressed state. There is often a small reduction in serum albumin with chronic starvation, although a level this low would not be expected.

6. *Patient A*. A triceps skinfold measurement at 20% of standard (about 3 mm) indicates extreme loss of fat reserves compatible with the status of patient A.

7. *Patient A*. In the absence of intervening stress, chronic energy deprivation results in a relatively well-adapted physiological state. Circulating levels of visceral proteins tend to be maintained near normal; metabolic rate and oxygen consumption are reduced; and protein losses are minimized (as reflected by a low rate of gluconeogenesis). In this situation the patient is more susceptible to nutritional complications of overzealous refeeding than to continued chronic inanition.

8. *Patient A*. As recognized by the noted physiologist Ancel Keys, the heart is more likely to go into failure during early recovery than during starvation. The heart muscle shrinks with starvation. With the introduction of carbohydrate, stimulation of insulin production increases renal sodium reabsorption and fluid retention. At the same time, the carbohydrate load stimulates catecholamine production and oxygen consumption and increases cardiac rate and cardiac output. The combination of volume expansion and cardiac demand predisposes to heart failure.

CASE STUDY 6   *Nutrition Assessment and Support*

1. *False*. Although the dietary intake pattern and the finding of perifollicular petechiae in this patient substantiate a diagnosis of scurvy, gum changes are only seen when teeth are present.

2. *True*. She has numerous findings that support the diagnosis of kwashiorkor: a predisposing history of poor protein intake accompanied by stress (in this case, surgical); clinical findings of widespread edema; easy, painless hair pluckability and a poorly healing surgical wound; and laboratory findings of reduced levels of serum albumin and lymphocytes.

3. *False*. Her present weight of 63 kg is spuriously high due to the edema. Based on her history of weight loss to 47 kg (her "ideal" weight), she is not now obese.

4. *True*. A low BUN does point toward a low recent intake of protein. When large and excessive amounts of protein are ingested, BUN rises, reflecting the increased rate of deamination and urea formation.

5. *False*. Based upon the 24-hour urinary excretion of urea nitrogen of 16 g per day, her estimated protein needs are 125 g per day (16 g + 4 g allowance for stool and nonurea urine nitrogen losses, multiplied by 6.25 to estimate protein from nitrogen).

6. *True*. Glucose is considered the fuel of reparation, since it is the only fuel that can be utilized by hypoxic tissues, young fibroblasts, and phagocytizing white blood cells. The need for glucose in the stressed state is a logical explanation for the increased rate of gluconeogenesis.

7. *False*. Despite the increased need for glucose in the stressed state, an exogenous source will help meet energy requirements but does not

effectively suppress endogenous glucose production, as would be expected in the fasting, nonstressed state.

8. *False*. Although a small proportion (about 10%) of our fat reserves are composed of essential fatty acids, this reserve may not be available if lipolysis is suppressed by the continuous infusion of glucose, as in this case. Intermittent, or cycled, parenteral alimentation will allow mobilization of stored essential fatty acids.

9. *True*. Intravenous dextrose solutions are made up of the monohydrous form of dextrose that contains 3.4 kcal/g. This is in contrast to dietary carbohydrate, which contains 4.0 kcal/g. Thus, 500 g dextrose × 3.4 kcal/g = 1700 kcal.

10. *True*. Zinc infused at a level of 2.5 mg per day would be expected to cover the needs of the stable adult. With the increased requirements due to infection and wound healing, intake should be increased in this case to at least 6 mg/day.

B

NORMAL LABORATORY VALUES

	Normal values
Hematology	
Hematocrit	
Men	39%-49%
Women	34%-44%
Hemoglobin	
Men	14-17 g/dl
Women	12-15 g/dl
Children	12-14 g/dl
Newborn	14.5-24.5 g/dl
Mean corpuscular volume	82-99 μ^3
Mean corpuscular hemoglobin	27-32 pg
Mean corpuscular hemoglobin concentration	32-36%
Platelets	150,000-400,000/mm^3
Reticulocytes	0.5%-1.5%
White blood cells	4000-11000/mm^3
Differential	
Lymphocytes	15%-52% (higher in children)
Neutrophils	35%-73% (lower in children)
Monocytes	2%-14%
Eosinophils	0%-5%
Basophils	0%-2%
Serum iron (Fe)	42-135 μg/dl
Transferrin	212-405 mg/dl
Iron-binding capacity	
Total, serum	270-400 μg/dl
% saturation	20%-55%
Serum ferritin	10-300 ng/ml
Iron deficiency	<10 ng/ml
Iron overload, chronic disease	Often >1000 ng/ml
Prothrombin time	70%-100% of control
Blood Chemistry	
Alkaline phosphatase	
1-3 mo	150-475 U/L
To 10 yr	120-320 U/L
Puberty	120-540 U/L
Adults	25-115 U/L

	Normal values

Blood Chemistry—cont'd

Ammonia (NH_3)	11-35 μmoles/L
Bilirubin	
Total	0-1.2 mg/dl
Direct	0.1-0.3 mg/dl
Calcium (Ca^{++})	8.5-10.5 mg/100 ml
Carbon dioxide content (HCO_3^-)	20-30 mEq/L
Carotene	79-233 μg/dl
Chloride	95-108 mEq/L
Creatinine	0.6-1.6 mg/dl
GGT (gamma glutamyl transpeptidase)	0-65 U/L
GOT (AST, aspartate aminotransferase)	7-40 U/L
Glucose, fasting	65-110 mg/dl
LDH (lactic dehydrogenase)	120-240 U/L
Magnesium (Mg^{++})	1.8-2.4 mg/dl
Osmolality	280-305 mOsm/kg plasma
Phosphorus	
Children	4.0-7.0 mg/dl
Adults	2.5-4.8 mg/dl
Potassium (K^+)	3.5-5.2 mEq/L
Proteins	
Total	6.4-8.4 g/dl
Albumin	3.5-5.5 g/dl
α_1 globulin	0.15-0.4 g/dl
α_2 globulin	0.5-0.9 g/dl
β globulin	0.7-1.1 g/dl
γ globulin	0.5-1.5 g/dl
Sodium (Na^+)	135-145 mEq/L
Urea nitrogen (BUN)	8-23 mg/dl

Urine Tests (24-hour excretion; varies with intake)

Calcium	30-250 mg (2-13 mEq)
Creatinine	800-1800 mg
Magnesium	150-300 mg (12-25 mEq)
Phosphorus	0.7-1.5 g
Potassium	0.8-3.9 (20-100 mEq)
Sodium	3-8 g (130-360 mEq)
Urea nitrogen (UUN)	See Table 10-4

Stool Tests

Fat	
Total	<6 g/24 hr (with dietary fat intake >50 g/day); <30% of dry weight
Neutral	1%-5% of dry matter
Free fatty acids	1%-10% of dry matter

	Normal values

Stool Tests—cont'd

Fat—cont'd

   Combined fatty acids   1%-12% of dry matter
     (as soap)

Nitrogen <2 g/24 hr or 10% of urinary nitrogen

Function Tests

D-xylose absorption test: Urine xylose 4-9 g/5 hr (or $>20\%$ of ingested
   after overnight fast, 25 g   dose); serum xylose 25-40 mg/dl 2 hr after
   xylose taken by mouth;   oral dose
   urine collected for fol-
   lowing 5 hr

Schilling test: Orally ad-   Excretion in urine of $>10\%$ of oral dose/24 hr
   ministered radio-labeled
   vitamin B_{12} following
   "flushing" parenteral injection of B_{12}; normaliza-
   tion of B_{12} excretion with
   exogenous intrinsic factor
   is diagnostic of intrinsic
   factor deficiency in patient with pernicious anemia and gastric atrophy

APPENDIX

C

DRUG-NUTRIENT INTERACTIONS*

DRUGS' EFFECTS ON NUTRIENTS

Drug	Nutrient effect
Antiinfective Agents	
Amikacin, gentamicin, sisomicin, and to- bramycin	Hypokalemia, hypomagnesemia, and hypocalcemia; increased uri- nary potassium and magnesium loss
Aminosalicyclic acid	Decreased vitamin B_{12} and fat absorption
Amphotericin B	Increased urinary excretion of potassium and decreased serum po- tassium and magnesium levels
Capreomycin	Hypokalemia, hypomagnesemia, and hypocalcemia
Cycloserine	Decreased serum folate
Isoniazid	Pyridoxine deficiency
Neomycin	Decreased absorption of carotene, iron, vitamin B_{12}, and choles- terol
Rifampin	Decreased serum 25-hydroxycholecalciferol level
Sulfasalazine	Folate deficiency
Anticoagulants	
Warfarin, indanedione derivatives	Decreased vitamin K–dependent coagulation factors
Cardiovascular Drugs	
Hydralazine	Pyridoxine deficiency

*Drug-nutrient interactions can manifest themselves in two ways, either from effects on nutritional status occurring as a result of drugs that have been prescribed or from altered effects of a drug as a result of dietary factors. The physician should be alert to the possibility of nutrient imbalances caused by medications so that undesired effects can be prevented or minimized and should also be aware of the effect food may have on the absorption of drugs so that the patient will receive maximum benefit from the drugs prescribed. However, in many cases, the significance of the nutrient effects is not well understood.

DRUGS' EFFECTS ON NUTRIENTS (continued)

Drug	Nutrient effect
Cardiovascular Drugs—cont'd	
Sodium nitroprusside	Decreased total serum vitamin B_{12}
Central Nervous System Drugs	
Aspirin	Decreased serum folate
	Decreased leukocyte and platelet ascorbic acid levels
Monoamine oxidase inhibitors	
Isocarboxazid	Increased sensitivity to tyramine-containing foods; possible development of hypertensive crisis
Pargyline	
Phenelzine	
Tranylcypromine	
Phenelzine	Pyridoxine deficiency
Tranylcypromine	
Phenobarbital	Decreased serum vitamin K_1
Phenytoin	Decreased serum folate, calcium, and 25-hydroxycholecalciferol levels
Electrolyte Drugs	
Potassium chloride, slow release	Decreased vitamin B_{12} absorption
Gastrointestinal Drugs	
Aluminum hydroxide	Decreased absorption of iron, phosphate, and vitamin B_{12}
Cholestyramine	Decreased absorption of vitamins A, D, E, K, B_{12}, and folate along with decreased absorption of inorganic phosphate and fat
Cimetidine	Decreased absorption of protein-bound vitamin B_{12}
Mineral oil	Decreased absorption of vitamins A, D, E, and K
Hormones	
Oral contraceptives	Decreased serum folate; pyridoxine deficiency; riboflavin deficiency
Other Agents	
Colchicine	Decreased absorption of vitamin B_{12}, sodium, potassium, fat, and nitrogen
Penicillamine	Pyridoxine deficiency

NUTRIENTS' EFFECTS ON DRUGS

Food can change the absorption characteristics of certain drugs. This can cause decreased effectiveness of the drug or can increase the absorption of the drug and result in a greater response to the drug or precipitate a side effect. Listed below are some of the drugs that can be affected by food, and instructions on how to minimize their effect on the drug.

Decreased Absorption (Avoid taking these drugs with food. Take at least 1 hour before or 2 hours after a meal.)

Penicillin G	Cephalexin	Levodopa/carbidopa	Zinc sulfate
Penicillin V	Methotrexate	Quinidine	Isoniazid
Cloxacillin	Tetracycline	Porpantheline	Iron
Ampicillin	Erythromycin stearate	Atenolol	

Increased Absorption (Food will alter the amount of the drug absorbed; therefore, the drug should be taken at the same time(s) each day relative to meals.)

Phenytoin	Propranolol
Carbamazepine	Dicumarol
Lithium	Sulfadiazine
Diazepam	Methoxsalen
Nitrofurantoin	Griseofulvin

Delayed Absorption (Food will delay the absorption of these drugs but not the overall amount absorbed. These drugs should be taken at least 1 hour before or 2 hours after a meal.)

Sulfisoxazole	Indomethacin
Suprofen	Ketoprofen
Aspirin	Cimetidine
Pentobarbital	Hydrochlorthiazide
Acetaminophen	Hydrocortisone
Tocainide	Doxycycline
Pentoxifylline	

Index

189